Stronger Legs & Lower Body

D1609433

TIM BISHOP

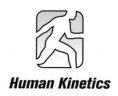

Human Kinetics

Library of Congress Cataloging-in-Publication Data

Bishop, Tim, 1964-
  Stronger legs & lower body / Tim Bishop.
      p. cm.
  ISBN-13: 978-0-7360-9295-1 (soft cover)
  ISBN-10: 0-7360-9295-1 (soft cover)
  1. Exercise. 2. Leg exercises. 3. Buttocks exercises. 4. Weight training.
  I. Title. II. Title: Stronger legs and lower body.
  GV508.B57 2012
  613.71--dc23

                              2011029050

ISBN-10: 0-7360-9295-1 (print)
ISBN-13: 978-0-7360-9295-1 (print)

Acquisitions Editor: Justin Klug; **Developmental Editor:** Carla Zych; **Assistant Editors:** Claire Marty and Derek Campbell; **Copyeditor:** Mary Rivers; **Graphic Designer:** Nancy Rasmus; **Graphic Artist:** Keri Evans; **Cover Designer:** Keith Blomberg; **Photographer (cover and interior):** Neil Bernstein; **Visual Production Assistant:** Joyce Brumfield; **Photo Production Manager:** Jason Allen; **Art Manager:** Kelly Hendren; **Associate Art Manager:** Alan L. Wilborn; **Illustrations:** © Human Kinetics; **Printer:** Versa Press

We thank Towson University in Towson, Maryland, and PerformFit Sports Performance and Fitness Training in Lutherville, Maryland, for assistance in providing the locations for the photo shoots for this book.

Human Kinetics books are available at special discounts for bulk purchase. Special editions or book excerpts can also be created to specification. For details, contact the Special Sales Manager at Human Kinetics.

Printed in the United States of America   10 9 8 7 6 5 4 3 2 1

The paper in this book is certified under a sustainable forestry program.

Human Kinetics
Website: www.HumanKinetics.com

United States: Human Kinetics
P.O. Box 5076
Champaign, IL 61825-5076
800-747-4457
e-mail: humank@hkusa.com

Canada: Human Kinetics
475 Devonshire Road Unit 100
Windsor, ON N8Y 2L5
800-465-7301 (in Canada only)
e-mail: info@hkcanada.com

Europe: Human Kinetics
107 Bradford Road
Stanningley
Leeds LS28 6AT, United Kingdom
+44 (0) 113 255 5665
e-mail: hk@hkeurope.com

Australia: Human Kinetics
57A Price Avenue
Lower Mitcham, South Australia 5062
08 8372 0999
e-mail: info@hkaustralia.com

New Zealand: Human Kinetics
P.O. Box 80
Torrens Park, South Australia 5062
0800 222 062
e-mail: info@hknewzealand.com

E5136

Contents

Introduction

People have been looking for ways to develop strength in the legs and lower body for over 2,000 years. Consider Milo of Croton, the wrestler who in the 6th century B.C. is said to have carried his baby calf every day until it was fully grown. As the calf slowly developed and gained size and strength, so did Milo. While our methods and understanding of resistance training have advanced since the time of Milo, people still strive to push their bodies to the limit in a quest for strength. And like Milo, people still use the principle of progressive resistance.

During the more than 25 years I have spent training, first as a professional athlete and then training others for professional sports, collegiate sports, strength development, mass development, and general health, I have seen firsthand the importance of a strong and stable lower body. It is the solid base from which other goals can be attained. I have seen this at the highest level of athletics right down to recreational golf. Hall of Famer and record-setting shortstop Cal Ripken is a fine example. In the off-season, he played very competitive basketball and performed strength training for the legs and lower body to keep his legs strong and powerful. His main focus, from a strength standpoint, was always legs and lower body, and he often told me how important his legs were in enabling him to stay competitive and perform at the highest level, day in and day out. His record of 2,632 consecutive major league baseball games suggests that he was doing something right! Of course, those who are not dedicated professional athletes have different goals and less time to devote to training. I've helped athletes at all levels achieve the type and degree of success they were seeking.

I wrote *Stronger Legs & Lower Body* to help you accomplish your goals, whatever they may be. Use the specific, progressive resistance exercises and programs to increase strength, and apply the advanced power development techniques and concepts to add challenge to your training. Use the variations to modify the exercises to suit your fitness level or to slightly alter the impact on the targeted muscles.

Think of this book as one that you can refer to often for guidance and direction as you plan and work through your training programs. Let it be your road map to training your legs and lower body. The exercises and programs will not only help you build a strong and stable base but will also have you looking and feeling better.

Stronger Legs and Lower Body is divided into three parts. Part I provides the background to help you understand the process of building strength. Part II contains complete descriptions of what I consider the best exercises for the lower body. Part III explains how to use programming to reach your goals, and it includes a variety of ready-made programs to suit particular target areas, methods of training, and time constraints.

To build strength, you must train hard on a consistent basis. The techniques and programs in this book will help you train effectively and efficiently so that you can reap the benefits that come from having stronger legs and a stronger lower body.

Exercise Finder

	MUSCLE TRAINING TARGETS						
	GLUTEAL EXERCISES						
Exercise	Glutes	Quads	Ham-strings	Low back	Stabi-lizing muscles	Core	Page
Body-weight squat	✓	✓					41
Barbell squat	✓	✓					42
Dumbbell squat	✓	✓					43
Smith press squat	✓	✓					44
Functional-trainer squat	✓	✓					45
Leg press	✓	✓					46
Walking lunge	✓	✓			✓	✓	47
Walking lunge with rotation	✓	✓			✓	✓	48
Bench single-leg squat	✓	✓					49
Step-up	✓	✓					50
Step-down	✓	✓					51
Single-leg press	✓	✓					52
4-way hip-machine extension	✓		✓				53
Ankle-weight standing hip extension	✓		✓				54
Ankle-weight all-fours hip extension	✓		✓				55
Miniband hip extension	✓		✓				56
Exercise-ball lying hip extension	✓			✓			57

Exercise	Glutes	Quads	Hamstrings	Low back	Stabilizing muscles	Core	Page
Double-leg bridge	✓		✓				58
Single-leg bridge	✓		✓				59
Miniband lateral walk	✓						60
Roman chair reverse hyperextension	✓		✓	✓			61
Sled push	✓	✓	✓	✓			62
Functional-trainer hip extension	✓		✓				63
Resistance-band hip extension	✓		✓				64

QUADRICEPS EXERCISES

Exercise	Quads	Glutes	Hamstrings	Hip flexors	Adductors	Abductors	Page
Barbell squat on weight plates	✓	✓					67
Front squat	✓	✓					68
Exercise-ball squat	✓	✓					69
Split squat	✓	✓	✓				70
Single-leg squat	✓	✓	✓				71
In-place lunge	✓	✓	✓				72
Weighted-sled walking lunge	✓	✓	✓				73
Walking retro lunge	✓	✓	✓				74
Drop lunge	✓	✓	✓				75
Lateral lunge	✓	✓	✓		✓		76

(continued)

Exercise	Quads	Glutes	Ham-strings	Hip flexors	Adduc-tors	Abduc-tors	Page
Slide lateral lunge	✓	✓	✓		✓	✓	77
Body-weight wide squat	✓	✓			✓		78
Straight-leg step-down	✓	✓	✓				79
Bench single-leg sit	✓	✓	✓				80
Machine leg extension	✓						81
Miniband low lateral walk	✓	✓				✓	82
Functional-trainer leg extension	✓						83
Functional-trainer straight-leg hip flexion	✓			✓			84
Manual-resistance leg extension	✓						85
Single-leg extension	✓						86
Wall sit	✓						87

HAMSTRING AND POSTERIOR CHAIN EXERCISES

Exercise	Ham-strings	Glutes	Quads	Hip flexors	Calves	Low back	Page
Trap-bar squat	✓	✓	✓		✓	✓	91
Straight-leg deadlift	✓	✓				✓	92
Good morning	✓	✓				✓	93
Romanian deadlift	✓	✓			✓		94

Exercise	Ham-strings	Glutes	Quads	Hip flexors	Calves	Low back	Page
Single-leg single-arm Romanian deadlift	✓	✓			✓	✓	95
Prone leg curl	✓	✓					96
Single-leg toe touch	✓	✓		✓	✓		97
Hamstring lower	✓	✓			✓		98
Double-leg straight-leg bridge	✓	✓			✓	✓	99
Single-leg straight-leg bridge	✓	✓			✓	✓	100
Double-leg flexed-leg bridge	✓	✓			✓	✓	101
Single-leg flexed-leg bridge	✓	✓			✓	✓	102
Roman chair hip extension	✓	✓				✓	103
Roman chair single-leg hip extension	✓	✓				✓	104
Prone negative leg curl	✓	✓					105
Manual-resistance prone leg curl	✓	✓					106
Functional-trainer leg curl	✓	✓					107
Exercise-ball supine leg curl	✓	✓			✓		108
Slide supine leg curl	✓	✓			✓		109
Prone single-leg curl	✓	✓					110

(continued)

LOWER-LEG EXERCISES						
Exercise	Gastroc-nemius	Soleus	Tibialis anterior	Tibialis posterior	Hip flexors	Page
Leg-press calf raise	✓					113
Leg-sled calf raise	✓					114
Standing calf raise	✓					115
Machine standing calf raise	✓					116
Functional-trainer standing calf raise	✓					117
Machine seated calf raise		✓				118
Seated calf raise		✓				119
Dynamic Axial Resistance Device (DARD) raise			✓			120
Resistance-band dorsiflexion			✓			121
Functional-trainer dorsiflexion			✓			122
Weight-plate seated dorsiflexion			✓			123
Heel walk			✓			124
Functional-trainer hip flexion with dorsiflexion			✓		✓	125
Standing dorsiflexion			✓			126
Resistance-band inversion			✓	✓		127

Exercise	Gastroc-nemius	Soleus	Tibialis anterior	Tibialis posterior	Hip flexors	Page
Resistance-band seated dorsiflexion			✓		✓	128

EXPLOSIVE MULTIJOINT EXERCISES

Exercise	Glutes	Quads	Ham-strings	Gas-troc-nemius and soleus	Erector spinae	Traps and delts	Page
Power clean	✓	✓	✓	✓		✓	132
Hang clean	✓	✓	✓	✓		✓	134
Power snatch	✓	✓	✓	✓		✓	136
Power jerk	✓	✓	✓	✓	✓	✓	138
Squat jump	✓	✓	✓	✓			139
Split squat jump	✓	✓	✓	✓			140
Vertical jump	✓	✓	✓	✓			141
Broad jump	✓	✓	✓	✓			142
Single-leg triple jump	✓	✓	✓	✓			143
Bench single-leg bounds	✓	✓	✓	✓			144

PART I

Training the Lower Body

CHAPTER 1

Lower-Body Anatomy

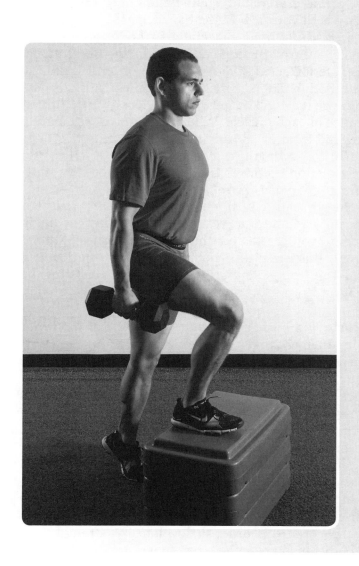

Understanding the anatomy of the lower body, particularly the muscle locations and their functions, will help you to get the most from the exercises and programs in this book. The muscles of the lower body work together to create a strong, stable base. Daily activities as well as athletics require the lower body to work in a synchronized manner; that is, while one muscle or muscle group is working, an opposing muscle or muscle group is supporting or stabilizing. Most muscles work in pairs called agonists and antagonists. During movement, the muscles responsible for moving a body part contract (shorten). These muscles are called agonists. The antagonist muscles work with the agonist muscles by elongating when the agonist shortens. The antagonist muscles return the body part back to the start position. A prime example of agonist and antagonist muscle groups in the lower body is the quads and the hamstrings.

In traditional weight training, and especially in bodybuilding, the muscles of the lower body are usually targeted individually. Recreational weightlifters usually isolate lower-body movements in order to gain size and simply look better. Bodybuilders, on the other hand, must isolate lower-body muscles because they will be judged very closely on definition and the overall appearance of each muscle. While these muscles generally work together, isolating and training specific muscles and muscle groups allow athletes to gain size and strength in specific areas.

The disadvantage of isolation exercises is that they are not very functional; they do not mimic everyday movements or athletic movements that generally require the muscles to bear weight and work as a unit. For example, the leg-extension machine is a great tool for isolating the quadriceps muscle, but because you are seated, thus not bearing weight, and moving at only one joint, this exercise is not very effective in developing functional strength. The front squat, on the other hand, calls for the muscles to bear weight and produce movement at three joints: ankles, knees, and hips.

In the chapters to come, the muscles and muscle groups of the lower body are discussed individually so that you can develop training programs for those areas. Unilateral and multijoint exercises are also included later in the book because they help create a strong, stable, and injury-free lower body. Sport performance and strength and conditioning coaches, as well as athletic trainers and physical therapists, often use unilateral and multijoint exercises to develop strength, speed, power, and balance for sports or to help in the prevention and recovery from injury. Unilateral and multijoint exercises are also a great way to add variety to your program.

This chapter offers an overview of the muscles of the quads, hamstrings, lower leg, glutes, and hip. It includes the names, locations, and functions of each muscle or muscle group and tells you how to target these individual muscles and muscle groups in order to develop size, strength, and muscle balance using body-weight exercises, machines, and free weights.

This chapter lays the foundation for applying all of the techniques you will learn throughout the rest of this book.

QUADRICEPS

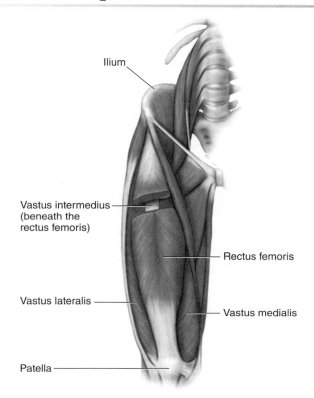

Ilium

Vastus intermedius (beneath the rectus femoris)

Vastus lateralis

Patella

Rectus femoris

Vastus medialis

Muscles Involved

The quadriceps, or quads, make up the anterior (forward) portion of the upper leg. The quad muscles support the body in a standing posture and are involved in extending the lower leg. The quads are composed of four muscles: *rectus femoris* (located in the middle of the thigh), *vastus medialis* (located on the medial side of the femur or the inner thigh), *vastus lateralis* (located on the lateral side of the femur or the outer thigh), and *vastus intermedius* (located between the vastus lateralis and the vastus medialis on the front of the femur). These four muscles are the largest and most powerful muscles of the body.

The main function of the quad group is to extend (straighten) the lower leg at the knee joint. The rectus femoris originates on the ilium of the pelvis and continues to the patella via the patellar tendon. The vastus lateralis originates on the greater trochanter, the vastus medialis originates on the medial surface of the femur, and the vastus intermedius originates on the anterior and lateral surfaces of the femur. These three muscles also continue on to the patella via the patellar tendon, which ultimately inserts into the tibial tuberosity.

The quad muscles make up about half of your body's overall muscle mass. Extension of the lower leg is very important for most sports. Bending, lunging, squatting, sprinting, and many other athletic movements also require leg extension. Strong and stable quads also help support the knee joint and assist in injury prevention.

Target Training

The quads are probably the easiest of the lower-body muscles to work because of the number of movements that can be made to extend the lower leg. Targeting individual quad muscles, however, can be a bit of a challenge. Generally, you can target different areas of the quads by changing foot placement or the angle of the feet.

For example, if you spread your feet slightly wider than normal and turn your toes out a few degrees more than usual during a squat exercise, you target the vastus medialis. Sometimes referred to as the teardrop due to its shape, the vastus medialis can also be targeted by performing a leg press with the feet set wide and slightly turned out on the platform. The leg-extension machine is another great way to target the vastus medialis, especially when extending the leg with the feet turned out slightly.

The vastus lateralis, or the outside of the thigh, can be targeted in much the same way as the inner quad. A narrow stance on a leg-press machine or a narrow stance during a front squat will target this area. The front squat will target the vastus lateralis because your weight is more forward than in a traditional back squat.

The vastus intermedius lies deep in the quad group, and it also extends the lower leg. Targeting this area is very similar to targeting the other three muscles. Squat, leg-press, and leg-extension exercises all target the vastus intermedius.

Performing negative, or eccentric, leg extensions targets the entire quad group much lower in the leg and closer to the insertion. Supine isometric leg raises are a great way to target the rectus femoris and are a safe alternative for those who have knee pain or knee injury.

HAMSTRINGS

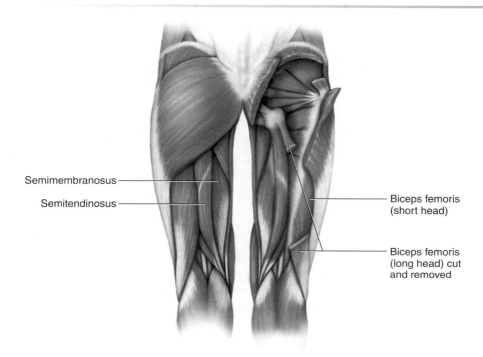

Semimembranosus

Semitendinosus

Biceps femoris
(short head)

Biceps femoris
(long head) cut
and removed

Muscles Involved

The hamstrings are made up of three muscles (and often include the associated tendons) located on the posterior thigh. The semitendinosus, semimembranosus, and biceps femoris are responsible for bending (flexing) the knee.

The biceps femoris has two (thus the name biceps) areas of origin. The longer head originates from the ischial tuberosity, and the short head originates from the linea aspera of the femur. The points of insertion for the two muscles are at the head of the fibula and the lateral condyle of the tibia. The semitendinosus originates on the ischial tuberosity and inserts on the proximal portion of the medial side of the tibia. The semimembranosus also originates on the ischial tuberosity and inserts on the medial condyle of the tibia.

You will notice that the hamstring group crosses the knee and the hip joint and therefore also assists with hip extension. The gluteus maximus also works with the hamstring group to help extend the hip. During walking or running, the hamstring group functions as an antagonist to the quads and acts as a decelerator of the lower leg. Along with the quads, the hamstrings help support the knee joint. Strong and flexible hamstrings, like strong quads, contribute to a strong stable base and help prevent injury by supporting the knee joint.

Target Training

The hamstrings are often overlooked when training for size and strength in the lower body. Stronger hamstrings will not only increase your hip and low back strength, but they will also give your legs a full, well-rounded appearance. You can target the hamstring muscles in one of two ways. The first is by doing exercises that require knee flexion. These include machine-based leg curls, exercise-ball leg curls, and manual-resistance leg curls. All three exercises involve movements that are made at the knee joint. The second way to target the hamstring group is by performing exercises that require hip extension. These exercises include straight-leg deadlifts, Romanian deadlifts, and single-leg toe touches. All three of these exercises work the hamstrings, with the hip as the dominant focus. Exercises that require knee flexion and exercises that require hip extension target the hamstring group in a slightly different manner.

Because of their proximity and shared function, it is impossible to isolate just one of the muscles of the hamstrings at any one moment. As with the quads, however, changing the angle of the foot placement on the floor (while performing free-weight exercises) or changing the angle of the foot placement on a platform or pad (while performing machine-based exercises) places greater emphasis on individual hamstring muscles. In a similar fashion, performing exercises with a slight bend in the knees puts greater emphasis on the upper hamstrings, while performing exercises with straight legs more effectively targets the lower hamstrings.

The biceps femoris lies on the posterior lateral aspect of the thigh. In addition to flexing the knee, it helps laterally rotate the thigh; therefore, if you turn your feet out slightly when performing leg curl movements, you target the biceps femoris more than the other two muscles. Both the semitendinosus and the semimembranosus lie on the medial aspect of the thigh. They flex the knee as well as medially rotate the thigh; to target these two muscles you can simply turn your feet slightly inward.

The hip-dominant movements target all three of the muscles in the hamstring group. You can target the lower portion of the semitendinosus, the semimembranosus, and the biceps femoris and the associated tendons by performing stiff-leg deadlifts or good-morning exercises. In these exercises, the knee joint remains stationary while the hip is moving. This places the emphasis on the insertion area. The upper portion of the hamstring group can be targeted by bending the knees slightly and performing Romanian deadlifts (RDL) or good mornings with the knees slightly bent. Doing an exercise-ball bridge (knees bent) also targets the proximal hamstrings during the hip extension movement of the exercise.

POSTERIOR LOWER LEG

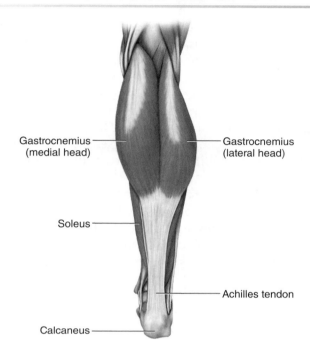

Gastrocnemius (medial head)

Gastrocnemius (lateral head)

Soleus

Achilles tendon

Calcaneus

Muscles Involved

The two main muscles of the posterior lower leg, or the calf, are the gastrocnemius and the soleus. The function of the gastrocnemius and the soleus is to lift or elevate the heel. This elevation of the heel, or plantar flexion, is critical in many athletic movements, especially sprinting. The soleus is called on for plantar flexion when the knee is bent and the gastrocnemius when the leg is extended.

The gastrocnemius is the largest and most visible of the two muscles. The soleus lies beneath the gastrocnemius and is much smaller. The gastrocnemius originates on the lateral and medial condyle of the femur and inserts on the posterior side of the calcaneus. The soleus originates on the posterior aspect of the fibula and the tibia and inserts on the calcaneus. Both of these muscles attach to the heel via the Achilles tendon.

Target Training

Targeting the calf muscles is much easier than targeting some other muscle groups of the lower leg. The two muscles (gastrocnemius and soleus) that make up the calf have very distinct functions and can therefore be targeted fairly easy. While the calf muscles may be easy to target, it is very difficult to increase size in this area.

The gastrocnemius is the larger of the two muscles and is more superficial. The two distinct heads originate from the posterior surfaces of the medial and lateral condyles of the femur. The gastrocnemius is targeted when the legs are straight. Therefore, exercises like the leg-press calf raise, standing calf raise, and machine standing calf raise are best for targeting this area of the calf.

The soleus, which lies deeper than the gastrocnemius, shares its insertion with the gastrocnemius to the calcaneus by way of the Achilles tendon. The soleus works with only one joint (the ankle) and is best targeted by exercises with the legs bent. Exercises like the seated calf raise and the machine seated calf raise are best for targeting this area of the calf.

ANTERIOR LOWER LEG

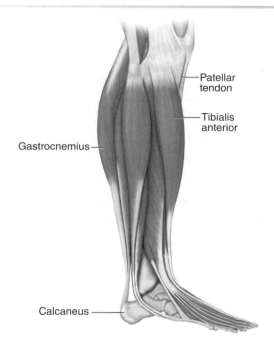

Patellar tendon

Tibialis anterior

Gastrocnemius

Calcaneus

Muscles Involved

The antagonist of the gastrocnemius and the soleus is the tibialis anterior. The tibialis anterior is responsible for dorsiflexion (flexing the ankle so that the toes move toward the shins) and inversion of the ankle. Dorsiflexion is an important movement for walking, jogging, and especially sprinting. The tibialis anterior also helps stabilize the ankle during foot contact with the ground. This muscle lies on the anterior portion of the lower leg on the lateral side of the tibia. Its actual origin is on the lateral condyle and body of the tibia, and its insertion is at the first metatarsal and first cuneiform of the foot.

Target Training

The tibialis anterior can be targeted by using the dynamic axial resistance device (DARD), a small piece of exercise equipment designed specifically for doing dorsiflexion, inversion, and eversion exercises or by doing resistance-band dorsiflexion or heel walking. Targeting the front part of the lower leg is just as important as targeting the back part of the lower leg. Proper muscle balance from front to back is important for preventing injury, especially in runners and those who perform other repetitive activities and are therefore prone to shin splints and similar injuries.

HIP MUSCULATURE

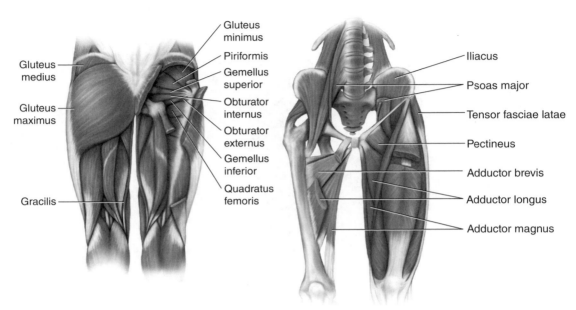

Gluteus minimus

Piriformis

Gemellus superior

Obturator internus

Obturator externus

Gemellus inferior

Quadratus femoris

Gluteus medius

Gluteus maximus

Gracilis

Iliacus

Psoas major

Tensor fasciae latae

Pectineus

Adductor brevis

Adductor longus

Adductor magnus

Muscles Involved

The hip joint is a very complex structure, and it serves many functions. Numerous muscles and muscle groups surround the hip joint and play various roles in movements of the thigh. The gluteal muscles work together to extend, rotate, and abduct the upper leg. Both the tensor fasciae latae and the glutes work to abduct the thigh. A group of six muscles, often referred to as the rotators, lie deep under the glutes and laterally rotate the thigh. The five muscles that move the thigh inward are commonly known as thigh adductors. The muscle groups that make up the hip musculature typically work in conjunction with one another to move the lower body in many planes.

The posterior muscles that help move the thigh are the gluteus maximus, the largest and most superficial of the three gluteal muscles; the gluteus medius; and the gluteus minimus. The gluteus maximus is a very strong muscle responsible for extending the leg and for external rotation. It originates in the lumbar region, on the ilium, sacrum, coccyx, and aponeurosis. The gluteus medius and the gluteus minimus lie beneath the gluteus maximus and work together to abduct the leg when it is in a neutral position, to externally rotate the thigh when the hip is flexed, and to internally rotate the thigh when the hip is extended. Both the gluteus medius and the gluteus minimus originate on the ilium and insert on the greater trochanter of the femur.

The tensor fasciae latae (positioned on the lateral surface of the hip) is, along with the gluteal muscles, a thigh abductor. The tensor fasciae latae originates on the anterior border of the ilium and iliac crest and inserts in the iliotibial tract.

The anterior muscles that move the thigh include the iliacus and the psoas major. The iliacus originates at the iliac fossa and inserts at the lesser trochanter of the femur. The psoas major originates at the transverse processes of the lumbar vertebrae. These two muscles work together to flex and rotate the thigh as well as flex the vertebral column.

Deep under the gluteus maximus lies a series of six lateral rotators of the thigh. They are the piriformis, gemellus superior, obturator internus, gemellus inferior, obturator externus, and quadratus femoris. These six very small muscles originate on the posterior aspect of the pelvis and attach to the head of the femur. These muscles are involved when the thigh is laterally rotated.

Finally, the group commonly known as the adductors consists of five medial muscles that move the thigh toward the midline of the body. The gracilis muscle is the most superficial, the pectineus is the most proximal, and the adductor longus is immediately lateral to the gracilis. The adductor brevis is located behind the adductor longus. The adductor magnus, the largest of the group, is on the medial side of the thigh. All five adductor muscles originate from different locations on the os pubis (pubic bone) and insert on the femur. The gracilis is the only one that inserts into the tibia. All five muscles assist with adduction, flexion, and rotation of the thigh.

Target Training

Targeting individual hip muscles is virtually impossible; however, targeting the hip and thigh muscle groups as a whole can be very easy. Squats, step-ups, and lunges all work the gluteal group very effectively. The 4-way hip machine (abduction movements) and the miniband lateral walk add resistance to the abduction movements of the thigh and target this area more specifically.

The iliacus and psoas major, which are primarily involved in hip flexion, may be targeted using retro lunges as well as the functional-trainer straight-leg hip flexion exercise. Lateral lunges work the adductor muscle group, which adducts and medially rotates the hip, as does the wide squat exercise. Exercises like the Romanian deadlift, single-leg toe touch, and exercise-ball hip extension work many of the muscles of the hip, both as primary movers and secondary stabilizers. All of these exercises also assist in building a stronger, more functional low back, in turn reducing the risk of low back injuries.

CHAPTER 2

Principles
of Training

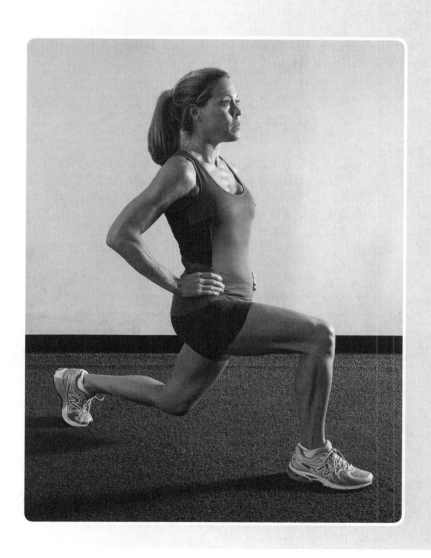

In any discipline, there are fundamentals, or principles, that must be followed to achieve success. Strength training is no exception. Without a basic knowledge of these fundamentals, you will never reach your goals. Training principles are the foundation of program design. These principles tell you the types and amounts of training that will produce specific effects so that you can choose workouts that will produce the results you're looking for. Certain training methods (high reps, low reps, high volume, and so on) can make a huge difference in physiological adaptations when it comes to a strength-training program. For example, high-volume training programs generally have a greater impact on body composition than lower-volume programs do. In the same way, the mode of training (type of equipment) may also influence certain neurological adaptations in different ways. Free-weight training will have a different impact than machine-based training.

The first part of this chapter explains the training principles behind the exercises and programs presented in this book. The second part looks at two other aspects of strength training that can make or break a program: form and technique.

OVERLOAD

Perhaps the most important principle of weight training is overload. Overload simply means providing a stimulus that is above and beyond the norm in order to trigger adaptation. If you overload your muscles, over time they become capable of handling a greater load and doing more work. This principle does not apply solely to weight training. Overloading flexibility or cardiorespiratory exercises also leads to adaptation and improvement in these areas.

There are several ways to accomplish weight-training overload. You can overload the body by increasing the training intensity, increasing the amount of weight used, increasing the number of exercises performed, and even decreasing the rest periods. Excessive loads cause minor trauma to the muscle fibers, which triggers a healing and strengthening response that, in turn, leads to increases in the size of the muscle fibers (hypertrophy).

Your muscles cannot tell the difference between body-weight exercises, resistance bands, free weights, and machines. As long as there is an overloading effect placed on the muscles, they will adapt and grow stronger. With that said, it would be hard for advanced weightlifters to overload their muscles using resistance bands because their muscles are already accustomed to such heavy loads. The stimulus required for creating an overload is unique to muscles and muscle groups as well as individuals. Those recovering from an injury may actually overload a muscle or muscle group with just a couple of pounds of resistance while a bodybuilder may need hundreds of pounds of resistance to overload the same muscle or muscle group. Regardless, the overload principle really comes down to hard work. If you are not continually striving to increase your effort through increased intensity, weight, or volume or through shortened rest periods, you will not improve.

SPECIFICITY

Specificity of training is often overlooked and frequently misunderstood. This principle simply implies that to improve at a particular exercise or skill, you must practice that exercise or skill. To improve a marathon time, a runner must run long distances; to get better at swimming, a swimmer must swim. A long distance runner does not reap the same benefits in her running ability from swimming as she does from her sport-specific training. And although swimming may have a place in a runner's program, to improve at running, a runner must run.

In terms of specificity, a resistance program should begin with general training and progress to very specific training. Beginners must perform very general exercises. Once they develop their strength base, their programs should include exercises designed more specifically to suit their goals. If an athlete wants to improve in the squat exercise, he needs to focus on squatting.

Other variables such as volume, load, and frequency of training must also be considered and adjusted according to individual goals. For example, to develop larger legs, the program should have more leg exercises than a program designed to develop strength. A program for someone who would like to develop endurance in the legs would include high repetitions with very little rest between sets.

INTENSITY

Training intensity is often thought of as the amount of weight that is being lifted. While this is one aspect of intensity, it does not quite describe the entire picture. You must also consider the number of repetitions performed. When you adjust the number of repetitions along with the amount of weight, you can maximize muscle recruitment to produce gains in size and strength.

Intensity is a relative term. What is intense for one person may be very easy for another. It will take some experimentation to find out what intensity of each exercise is best for you based on your goals.

Training at full intensity refers to lifting the heaviest weight you can for as many reps as you can manage. This controversial method, sometimes referred to as lifting to muscle failure, or high-intensity training, is used to gain strength and size, but there is little good research to support it. Training to failure on a regular basis may be counterproductive; it increases the risk of injury both acutely (because of the extreme effort during each lift) and chronically (because of the maximum effort given workout after workout).

It is not necessary to train at maximum intensity on a regular basis. You can achieve size and strength by training with higher volumes of exercises at a moderate to heavy load. You may want to consider using high-intensity training to shake things up and add variety to your overall program, but I would not recommend using it for long periods.

When you perform multiple sets of an exercise and multiple exercises per session, lifting to failure can be very fatiguing. If you are truly training to failure, assuming you are using the same weight in each set, the number of reps you can complete during each set will decline. Furthermore, as you progress into your lifting session for the day, you will find less energy for the exercises that you perform later in the workout. While this is true with any type of training, training to failure will show this even more. Make sure you mix up the order of your lifts in order to create muscle balance throughout your body.

VOLUME

Training volume refers to the amount of load (the amount of work) that is performed during a training session. In other words, it is a function of the number of exercises, broken down into sets and reps, completed in a workout session; it can also refer to the number of sets and reps performed for a given muscle or muscle group. Higher volumes with moderate loads are considered the best for hypertrophy training (increasing size), while lower volumes with higher loads are best for pure strength gains.

If you are interested in gaining size, you should try to complete approximately 4 to 6 exercises per muscle or muscle group for 3 sets of 8 to 12 repetitions per exercise (not including warm-up sets). This adds up to about 12 to 18 total sets for each muscle or muscle group per training session. Again, these sets should be performed with moderate loads.

If your goal is to gain strength, you would complete a fewer number of sets and reps. For strength gains, you should perform 2 to 4 exercises per muscle or muscle group, completing 2 or 3 sets of 1 to 6 repetitions per exercise (not including warm-up sets). Remember, for pure strength you should be using heavy loads with plenty of rest between exercises as well as between training sessions. Full muscle recovery after training with heavy loads is the key to gaining strength.

DURATION

We usually think of the duration of exercise in relation to cardiorespiratory exercise. We are told that we should do 20 to 40 minutes of aerobic exercise on a regular basis. However, duration is a factor in weight training as well. In weight-training duration refers to both the duration, or length of time, of each exercise session and the duration of the entire program.

The length of time it takes to complete any one particular weight-training session depends on several factors, including the amount of time it takes you to set up and adjust equipment (putting on and taking off weight plates, changing pins, levers, and so on), the time you spend talking with others around you, and the prescribed rest periods. You should always take these factors into account when designing your workouts. Unilateral exercises will also take longer because they require exercising one side of the body at a time. Generally, strength-based programs take longer than endurance-based programs because of the longer rest periods needed in a pure strength program.

You should also monitor the length of time you spend in any one given program—that is, the length in days, weeks, and months. Generally it is beneficial to make changes in your program about every six weeks, although the ideal time period depends on your ability level, your time devoted to training, and your training goals. Following a given program for too long may lead to a plateau in your training as well as physical overtraining and boredom.

FREQUENCY

Training frequency refers to the number of sessions that you train a muscle or muscle group during a specific period (usually one week). The correct training frequency depends on many factors; intensity, volume, fitness level, time allotted, and training goals all factor into how many sessions you will train per week. Training sessions that include heavy weights, intense negatives (exercises in which great emphasis is put on the eccentric phase of the lift to prepare the muscles to handle heavier loads), and multijoint exercises tend to require longer recovery times between sessions. Generally, if you train your entire body in one session, you will need at least two days off before repeating that same workout. On the other hand, if you do a split routine that works the upper body one day and the lower body the next, or that alternates specific muscles or muscle groups, you can work out two days back to back and then take one day off before repeating the two-day sequence again. In either scenario, you need to allow the muscles to recover fully before training them again. Your particular goals will dictate which routine is best for you. If you want increased strength, two days of rest between sessions is probably best. If you want to become leaner and lose body fat or achieve muscle endurance, a split routine that allows you to train more often and burn more calories is probably a better option.

OVERTRAINING

Overtraining is not a principle of training, but it is a very important concept to be aware of when developing your program. Overtraining refers to training too much without proper regeneration periods. Proper weight-training programs are based on acute stress on the body followed by periods of recovery or regeneration. If a program does not allow for adequate recovery, the stressors remain and become chronic. Stress hormones, when left unchecked for long periods, can lead to changes in resting heart rate, blood pressure, and respiration patterns along with various other physiological changes. This chronic stress may negatively affect the muscular, skeletal, cardiovascular, and endocrine systems.

Overtraining not only results in a drop in performance, but it can also make you weaker. Fatigue and weakness from overtraining may also lead to a suppressed immune system as well as injury to the muscles and joints.

Symptoms of overtraining may include general fatigue, decreased body weight and appetite, and increased muscle soreness and resting heart rate. If you notice signs of overtraining, decrease the frequency, intensity, and duration of exercise until you feel better.

You can prevent overtraining by increasing your intensity and duration gradually as well as periodizing your workout schedule. Chapter 3 includes various split-routine options you can use to train hard without overtraining. Proper nutrition, hydration, stress-management strategies, and rest also help prevent overtraining.

PROPER FORM AND TECHNIQUE

Throughout the exercise section of this book you will notice instructions that relate to posture, specific joint movements (such as extending, flexing, and descending), foot placement, tempo, and breathing. These aspects of strength training are often overlooked, but they have a significant impact on the effectiveness of a strength program and, more important, the risk of injury.

Posture and Joint Movements

Maintain good posture, especially in the spinal region, when you squat, lunge, or step. Keeping your back straight (not rounded), your shoulders drawn back, and your pelvis in a neutral position allow you to handle heavier resistances without compromising your spine. When you lunge or step, keep your knees at 90 degrees to prevent the knees from moving out over the toes. Keep your body weight evenly distributed throughout your feet or even slightly back toward your heels. The combination of limiting knee flexion to 90 degrees and keeping the weight distribution toward the heel takes the pressure off your patellar tendon and the knee joint itself.

Execute machine-based exercises correctly and carefully, too. Proper posture during a leg-press exercise is just as important as proper posture during a squat. Keep your back flat against the pad of the machine and drive the platform with your feet flat, keeping your weight toward the middle of your foot. Limiting the amount of flexion during a leg-extension exercise on a machine protects your tendons and joints just as keeping your knee at 90 degrees during a lunge exercise does.

Foot Placement

Foot placement is addressed in almost every lower-body exercise in this book because where you place your feet on the floor or on the machine will functionally change the exercise. Pay close attention to the width (distance apart) of your foot placement and the direction of the toes (pointed out, in, or straight ahead). Generally speaking, widening your stance and turning your feet outward place greater stress on the inner portion of the thigh. Turning the feet inward is usually performed on machine-based exercises only, such as those on a leg-extension machine, and places a greater emphasis on the outer portion of the thigh.

Tempo

Tempo refers to the pace at which you go through each movement in the exercise. How many times have you seen someone in a gym race through an exercise with his entire body rocking in order to generate enough momentum to move the weight? Racing through an exercise often compromises technique and increases the risk of injury. There are times when a faster pace is appropriate, such as when training for explosive power; however, for the most part, a slow, controlled movement is best.

An exercise has two actions or phases of movement: the concentric phase, or the shortening of the muscle (often referred to as the exertion portion of the exercise); and the eccentric phase, or the lengthening of the muscle (often referred to as the negative or resisting portion of the exercise). During a squat, for example, the eccentric phase occurs during the part of the movement when the hips, knees, and ankles are flexing and the weight is being lowered. The concentric phase occurs when the hips, knees, and ankles extend, pushing the weight back up to the starting position. The tempo is the rate at which you move during both the concentric and eccentric phases of the repetition. It's the speed of the movement.

Depending on your goals, it may be advantageous to favor a slightly quicker tempo or a slightly slower tempo. Generally, it is important to control the weight. A slow, controlled lift is usually the safest and most effective way to perform an exercise. A general rule would be to lower the weight (eccentric movement) at a pace of about 2 to 4 seconds and to lift or push the weight at a pace of about 1 to 3 seconds. The soreness you often feel from resistance training is usually the result of the negative, or eccentric, portion of the lift. While there are some lifting techniques that are ballistic in nature (for instance, power cleans) and require a very fast tempo, generally speaking, a controlled lift with good technique is best.

Breathing

Proper breathing is an important part of weight training. Often people hold their breath while lifting weights, mistakenly thinking that this gives them more power. Inhaling brings oxygen into the lungs and allows it to be transported throughout the body via blood cells. Exhaling rids the body of toxins such as carbon dioxide. Proper breathing during exercise oxygenates the working muscles, supplies them with nutrient-rich blood, and prevents the buildup of the waste products.

You have probably heard that you should breathe in during the concentric (shortening) phase of the lift and breathe out during the eccentric (lengthening) phase of the lift. Breathing out during the entire eccentric phase, however, is not the most effective procedure.

The proper way to breathe during a lifting exercise is to exhale during the work (push) phase and to inhale during the recovery (rest) phase. In the leg-press exercise, for example, inhale just before you exert force with your feet on the platform. As you exert the force and push the weight of the platform, exhale.

For healthy people with no heart or blood pressure conditions, a modified version of the Valsalva maneuver is a safe and effective way to lift heavy loads. This maneuver involves holding your breath against a closed windpipe and exerting pressure. This procedure was named for Valsalva, a 17th-century physician who studied the human ear and esophagus. Let's apply the modified Valsalva maneuver to the squat exercise. Once you have the bar on your back, expand your chest with your head and neck in a neutral position. Take a deep breath down into your belly and then begin to descend with the weight. Hold your breath through the bottom of your descent and then begin to breathe out *after* you push through the sticking point of the lift on the ascent. The intra-abdominal pressure that is built by holding in your breath helps support your spine while holding the heavy load. Note that if you have high blood pressure or any heart conditions, you should talk with your physician before attempting any weight-training program, and you should not use the modified Valsalva method.

CHAPTER 3

Exercise Planning

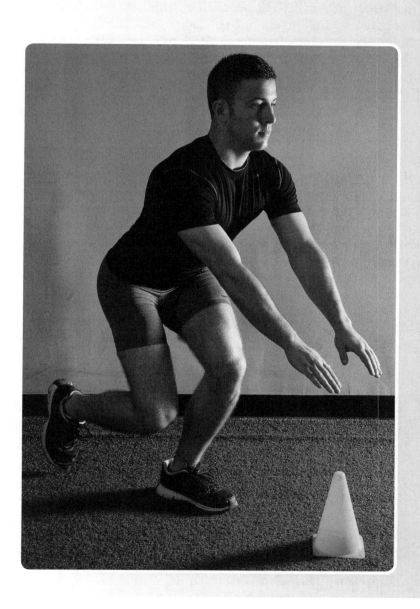

When you design your workout program, you must consider how many sets and reps you will perform, how much weight you will use, how much rest you will have in between reps and sets, what type of equipment or lifts you will use or do, and how many days per week you will train. You should also consider looking at the big picture and deciding how many months of the year you will stay on any given program. This concept is periodization. Periodization is the process of monitoring and changing up your workouts to keep them fresh and effective. If you repeatedly do the same workout, your body will adapt to this program, and you simply will not progress any further. Setting up distinct training periods shocks your body, giving it new challenges that will help you continue to make strength and fitness gains. There are many ways to change up a routine. Manipulating the sets, reps, resistance, rest periods, order of exercise, types of exercises, and so on allows for an infinite number of combinations that you can use to bring change to your program.

TRAINING CYCLES

Typical periodized programs can be divided into three basic time periods, or cycles, each of which encompasses a particular period and has specific objectives. The first is a macrocycle. This cycle is the big picture of your overall program; it has a long cycle, often covering one year. This is especially applicable for athletes as they prepare for a performance season. The mesocycle is a medium-length period within the macrocycle with several phases. A mesocycle typically lasts from 6 weeks to several months. A microcycle is a very short period within a mesocyle. This cycle is often measured by what you will do in one particular week or even as little as one day. The length of each phase will differ depending on your goals and time available for training.

Macrocycles and mesocycles have multiple phases within them. The following four phases, as they are described, can be considered mesocycles within a larger macrocycle.

The first of the four phases is a *preparation phase*, when you are preparing the body for a more intense phase to follow. This phase is very general and involves low volume and low intensity. It may last anywhere from 4 to 6 weeks.

The second phase within a cycle is the *strength-building phase*. This phase builds the base, or foundation, for the remaining phases. It usually involves a moderate to high volume with moderate intensity. The strength-building phase can last 12 to 24 weeks.

The third phase within a cycle is the *strength and power phase*. This phase is the most intense phase. It is a time of building pure strength and power. The strength and power phase involves moderate volume but very high intensity. This phase may last anywhere from 4 to 8 weeks.

The last is a *maintenance phase*. This phase is used to maintain the gains that you made during the previous phases. The volume should be low, but the intensity should be high. This phase is often misunderstood. Many people think that a maintenance phase is low volume and low intensity. But you must keep your intensity high in order to maintain your strength and power gains.

After you have completed your macrocycle, you should enter a time of recovery or active rest. This is a time to allow your body to heal and regenerate. This is not a time to do nothing but rather a time to participate in lower-intensity activities while allowing your body the time it needs to rest in preparation for your next macrocycle. The duration of this recovery period depends on your goals, and if you're an athlete, how long your off-season is.

Sample Periodized Plan for Maximum Strength

All good training programs should start with the end, the final goal, in mind. Using the goal to set the overall timeline, manipulate sets and reps within each cycle or phase to suit your specific goals. For example, an athlete who would like to reach peak strength by early the next summer would begin a preparation phase in the fall. This phase would be low intensity (50 to 60 percent of the 1-repetition max) and moderate volume (1 to 3 sets of 10 to 12 repetitions). The strength-building phase would follow in the late fall or early winter. This phase would have moderate intensity (60 to 75 percent of the 1-repetition max) and moderate to high volume (2 to 4 sets of 8 to 12 reps). This portion of the cycle takes the longest (12 to 24 weeks) because of the time involved for the body to adapt to the increased volume and intensity and to begin to increase muscle mass. The strength and power phase would begin in early to mid-spring. This phase would be marked by high intensity (80 to 95 percent of 1-repetition max) and low volume (2 to 3 sets of 1 to 6 reps after a warm-up set). Over the course of the strength and power phase, the neuromuscular response would improve, increasing motor unit recruitment and muscle activation, thus allowing the athlete to reach maximum strength by early summer.

REPS

In chapter 2 we talked about reps and how they relate to your particular goals. You recall that, in general, you would choose low reps (3 to 6) and high resistance for strength gains, slightly higher reps (8 to 12) and moderate to heavy resistance for muscle size, and a high rep range (15 to 20) with low to moderate resistance for muscular endurance. Let's take a look at each one of these goals.

1. **Muscular strength:** Strength is the ability to move or lift a maximum amount of weight one time. Max deadlifts and squats are examples of exercises that demand pure strength. The method for developing strength, then, is to overload the muscles with very heavy weights. To reach this heavy overload, you must keep the number of reps low. The ideal number of reps for loading the muscles to near max is 3 to 6 per set. Performing too many reps will fatigue the muscles prematurely. Higher numbers of reps are not as effective in building strength. Your muscles, tendons, and ligaments also need to adapt to these heavy loads to gain overall strength.

2. **Muscle size (hypertrophy):** Muscle strength and size go hand in hand. As you increase your strength, you increase your size. However, if your focus is mainly on developing size, then you need a high-volume, moderate-rep range (8 to 12), along with moderate to high intensity. The higher volume of work demanded by this scenario best promotes muscle growth. However, this is not black and white. You can favor the strength side of a hypertrophy program by doing 6 to 8 reps and obtain the benefits of both strength and size gains.

3. **Muscular endurance:** Muscular endurance is the ability of your muscles to perform repeated bouts of work. Swimmers, runners, and cyclists would all benefit from a program with a higher range of reps (15 to 20). Muscular endurance programs are also great for those just learning how to weight train. Using lighter weights allows you to work on proper form, whereas starting with heavier weights can lead to poor technique and subsequent injuries.

One fallacy that I hear very often is that in a maintenance program (especially with in-season athletes) you only need to do lighter weights and higher reps to maintain your strength. This is simply not true. Programs with high numbers of reps and low intensity will develop muscular endurance but are not optimal for the maintenance of strength gains.

Many people use differing ranges of rep numbers for different muscles or muscle groups. Most people, for example, train the calves with a relatively high number of reps and the quads with lower to moderate numbers of reps. Regardless of your goals, it is very important to change your rep ranges throughout your program. Your body adapts to doing the same number of reps and amount of weight over time. A combination of the three ranges (3 to 6, 8 to 12, and 15 to 20) over the course of a year-long cycle is probably ideal.

REST PERIODS

The amount of time you rest between sets depends on your specific training goals as well as the types of exercises that you are performing. For instance, performing compound exercises requires periods of rest longer than those needed for isolation movements. Complex training also requires longer rest periods between pairs of exercises. Longer rest periods are necessary because of the amount of work that is being done in these two instances. If your goal is to increase strength, a longer rest period between sets is best. The heavier loads necessary for strength gains may require 2 to 5 minutes of rest in order to fully recover before repeating another set. When you are training for muscular endurance, very little rest between sets is required. A short rest (about 30 seconds) is adequate. Do not rest any longer than this if your goal is to develop muscular endurance, because any rest periods longer than 30 seconds will not be effective.

The length of hypertrophy rest periods falls in between the lengths for rest periods when training for muscular strength and those when training for muscular endurance. Allow proper recovery time so that you can lift the moderate to heavy loads with greater volume; however, you do not want to fully recover because you want to fatigue the muscles, encouraging them to grow. A proper rest period for hypertrophy training is in the 60- to 90-second range.

DYNAMIC WARM-UP AND FLEXIBILITY WORK

Many people who exercise and play sports often confuse stretching with warming up. But there is a very distinct difference between warming up and stretching. A warm-up of some sort is much more important than stretching. In fact, you can make an argument that stretching is not necessary before your lifting program. The purpose of your preexercise warm-up routine should be to elevate your heart rate and increase the temperature of your muscles, tendons, ligaments, and joints. You simply can't do these things with a cold, static stretch routine.

A general warm-up, such as light jogging on a treadmill, riding a stationary bike, or doing a stair stepper, is a good start. Any of these activities will increase your heart rate and begin the warm-up process necessary for preparing your body for the more intense exercise to follow. Five minutes is probably enough time to spend on the general warm-up. Spending too much time here will compromise the quality of your strength program.

Follow the general warm-up with an active, or dynamic, warm-up routine. Movements like leg swings, walking lunges, and over–under hurdle walks are great ways to increase your range of motion in and around your joints and muscles. The active warm-up should last about 5 minutes; the entire preweight warm-up routine should take no longer than 10 minutes.

The final stage of your warm-up routine should be a light weightlifting warm-up. Always do a lighter warm-up set before the first set of your lead-in exercise. Although individual needs vary, generally 1 set of 10 to 12 repetitions at a weight that is about 50 to 60 percent of your prescribed weight for the next lift should suffice. For example, if you are planning on doing 3 sets of squats, 10 reps each, as your first exercise of the day, begin with a set of light squats first and do not count it as your first set. Once you complete your squats, it will not be necessary to perform a warm-up set for each additional exercise that you perform.

If you switch muscle groups (moving to leg curls, for example), you may need a warm-up set of this exercise before moving on to your set and rep plan for the day. If you just performed multijoint exercises, which involve most muscle groups of the lower body, you probably do not need a warm-up set.

Postworkout stretching is great for cooling down and helping to maintain flexibility. This is the time for additional static stretching if you would like to work on your range of motion or decrease the amount of stiffness you may get from your workout.

TRAINING SPLIT DESIGNS

It's time to put your program together. A training split is the system you use to schedule your week's training by planning the number and type of training sessions you do throughout the week. The type of split you choose determines what your weekly lifting schedule looks like. You need to design your program based on your goals and the time available to you to train.

Begin with deciding how many days per week you can devote to each muscle group. You should plan on working each muscle group one or two times per week if your goal is size and strength, and three times per week if your goal is muscular endurance. Once you determine how many days per week you can train, you must decide how long you can train in each session as well as which muscle groups you prefer to pair up. Muscle groups are paired and split so that some muscles are resting while others are working. The following are examples of typical splits.

■ **Whole-body split** (3 times per week). In the whole-body split routine, you train all of your muscle groups in one session. For example, you would train Monday, Wednesday, and Friday, or Tuesday, Thursday, and Saturday. You must have one full day of recovery between sessions. The biggest advantage of this type of routine is that you only have to go to the gym three days per week. This is ideal for those who have a limited schedule. The disadvantage is that you must spend a very long time in

TABLE 3.1 **Whole-Body Training Split**

Day	Muscle groups trained
Monday	Legs, chest, back, shoulders, biceps, triceps, core
Tuesday	Off
Wednesday	Legs, chest, back, shoulders, biceps, triceps, core
Thursday	Off
Friday	Legs, chest, back, shoulders, biceps, triceps, core
Saturday	Off
Sunday	Off

the gym on those training days. The volume of exercises that you need to perform in this program will take a lot of time. If you must, you can limit your rest times in order to speed up your workouts. Table 3.1 shows you an example of a whole-body split routine.

■ **Two-day split** (2 or 3 times per week for each muscle group). The two-day split allows you to train each muscle group up to three times in a week. Splitting the entire body in half over two days shortens your workouts compared to the whole-body split. The two-day split keeps you in the gym up to six days per week, but it also shortens the length of each session. If your goal is strength, then you can use the standard two-day split, putting you in the gym only four days per week rather than six. Feel free to do your core exercises on any or all of your workout days. Table 3.2 shows you an example of a standard two-day split.

TABLE 3.2 **Two-Day Training Split**

Day	Muscle groups trained
Monday	Legs, back, biceps, core
Tuesday	Chest, shoulders, triceps
Wednesday	Off
Thursday	Legs, back, biceps
Friday	Chest, shoulders, triceps, core
Saturday	Off
Sunday	Off

How you split up your exercises is up to you. Just make sure you are not working the same muscle groups on back-to-back days. Another easy example of designing a two-day split is to separate your upper body from your lower body. Do all upper-body exercises on one day and all of your lower-body exercises on the next. You can do core exercises on the days where you feel they fit best for you. An example of the upper–lower two-day split can be seen in table 3.3.

TABLE 3.3   Upper–Lower Two-Day Training Split

Day	Muscle groups trained
Monday	Chest, back, shoulders, biceps, triceps, core
Tuesday	Legs
Wednesday	Off
Thursday	Chest, back, shoulders, biceps, triceps
Friday	Legs, core
Saturday	Off
Sunday	Off

■ **Three-day split** (1 or 2 times per week for each muscle group). A three-day split routine trains the entire body but spreads it out over a three-day period. If your goals are to train each muscle group one time per week, you will have only three workout sessions per week. If you would like to focus on each muscle group twice per week, you will have to double the total number of workouts to six for the week. One common way to break down the three-day split routine is to divide the upper-body training into two workouts and leave the lower body for a day of its own. You can divide the upper-body training into two sessions by working the pushing muscles (chest, shoulders, triceps) on one day and the pulling muscles (back and biceps) on another day. The push–pull routine allows that day's unused muscles to recover while the upper body is being trained. Table 3.4 shows an example of a push–pull–legs three-day split, and table 3.5 shows a second option for a three-day split.

TABLE 3.4 Push–Pull–Legs Three-Day Training Split

Day	Muscle groups trained
Monday	Chest, shoulders, triceps
Tuesday	Back, biceps
Wednesday	Legs
Thursday	Off
Friday	Repeat Monday if goal is 2 times per week
Saturday	Repeat Tuesday if goal is 2 times per week
Sunday	Repeat Wednesday if goal is 2 times per week

TABLE 3.5 Standard Three-Day Training Split

Day	Muscle groups trained
Monday	Chest, back
Tuesday	Legs
Wednesday	Biceps, triceps, shoulders
Thursday	Off
Friday	Repeat Monday if goal is 2 times per week
Saturday	Repeat Tuesday if goal is 2 times per week
Sunday	Repeat Wednesday if goal is 2 times per week

■ **Four-day split** (once a week for each muscle group). The four-day split trains your entire body over a four-day period. The short training sessions make this routine ideal for training with heavy volume. Feel free to pair your exercises in any combination that you like. The built-in off days give you flexibility in case your schedule does not permit a workout on a certain day. You can always lift back-to-back days if needed. Table 3.6 shows an example of a four-day split routine.

TABLE 3.6 **Four-Day Training Split**

Day	Muscle groups trained
Monday	Chest, back
Tuesday	Off
Wednesday	Legs
Thursday	Shoulders
Friday	Off
Saturday	Biceps, triceps
Sunday	Off

■ **Five-day split** (once a week for each muscle group). The five-day training split allows you to train the entire body over a period of five days. This sequence allows you to focus on each muscle group with as much volume as you would like. The combinations of pairings and exercises are almost endless with this format. Table 3.7 shows you one example of a five-day split.

TABLE 3.7 **Five-Day Training Split**

Day	Muscle groups trained
Monday	Chest, triceps
Tuesday	Back
Wednesday	Legs
Thursday	Off
Friday	Shoulders
Saturday	Biceps
Sunday	Off

PAIRING MUSCLE GROUPS

When you design your program, you should follow two guidelines. First, always perform exercises for the larger muscle group before exercises for the smaller muscle group. For instance, you do not want to work your calves before squatting. You will need all of your strength to devote to the squat. Fatiguing a smaller muscle group (like the calves) before working the larger muscle group (like the quads and glutes) will inhibit the strength gains that you want from the squat, and it can also be dangerous. Performing a squat when your legs are tired is unsafe.

Second, if you have identified weaknesses in certain muscle groups, try to make them a priority in your program. Do the lifts that involve these weaker areas first. This keeps these weaker areas fresh and able to work harder, allowing the weaker areas to catch up. You might also consider adding more volume to the muscle groups that you are trying to improve. If you have identified one muscle group as very weak, you can devote one entire session each week to just that muscle group. This allows you to spend more time on this area with fresh, fully rested muscles.

TYPES OF EXERCISES

When you are training a muscle or muscle group, you would typically perform 3 to 5 sets of 3 to 5 different exercises. By using differing modes (body weight, free weights, machines, and so forth) of exercise, you are able to work the muscle or muscle group in a variety of motions, angles, and intensities. This variety allows you to maximize the stress that is being placed on the muscle. In chapters 4 through 8 you will learn about specific exercises for each lower-body muscle group. The following paragraphs, however, break those exercises into categories. All of the exercises in this book fall into one of the following.

Free-Weight Exercises

Performing free-weight exercises should be the ultimate goal of anyone who wants to increase strength. There are two basic types of free weights: barbells and dumbbells. Barbells are typically 5- to 7-foot-long bars (1.5 to 2.1 m) with weights that can be loaded on the ends; dumbbells are individual weights held in the hand. Exercises performed with barbells and dumbbells allow for greater recruitment of stabilizing muscles (secondary muscles that assist the primary muscle) and allow a greater range of motion. Both barbells and dumbbells give you the opportunity for greater strength gains, and exercises using them assist with injury prevention. Many machines have cables, pulleys, weight stacks, cams, and rods that often affect the true amount of weight that is being lifted. Using free weights provides a more accurate measure of your strength. A 20-pound weight is a 20-pound weight. Dumbbells are also a great way to balance out your body's weaknesses. The use of single limbs when using dumbbells allows any undertrained muscles to catch up with the others, creating greater overall muscle balance.

Machine-Based Exercises

Machine-based weight-training exercises are a great supplement to free-weight exercises. Machines are generally very safe and can usually be used without a spotter present. While machines limit the number of stabilizing muscles that are recruited, they allow you to push or pull harder without worrying about having to balance the weight. This, in turn, helps you over-load the target area more easily. The Smith press machine is an excellent example of this. You can squat heavier loads without having to maintain your balance as you would with a barbell on your back.

Cables are another effective means of overloading muscles throughout a full range of motion. For instance, in the cable hip-abduction exercise the cable allows a full range of motion with constant resistance through various directions. Because of this, cables are great for mimicking sport performance training movements as well as for rehabilitative exercises. Machine-based exercises are a safe alternative to free weights, and they also add variety to your program. In fact, some muscle groups are more challenging to train using only free weights. For instance, the number of free-weight movements capable of working the hamstring group is limited. By adding a variety of leg curl machines and cables, you can add a greater volume of exercises for this area.

Unilateral and Bilateral Exercises

You can perform most lower-body exercises using a single leg (unilaterally) versus using both legs (bilaterally). You can use your body weight, dumb-bells, weighted vests, and even machines to perform unilateral lower-body exercises. For example, you can do a unilateral leg-press movement simply by using a weight that is lighter than you would use bilaterally. Do a single-leg squat with your body weight, or you can add a weighted vest to make it more challenging. Unilateral training is a great way to challenge your body by adding variety as well as allowing you to lift more weight on a limb that might be weaker than the other. Lower-body unilateral training is also great for overall stability and balance.

Compound and Isolation Exercises

A compound exercise is one that involves multiple joints throughout the movement. There are many examples of compound exercises, especially when it comes to the lower body. The squat, lunge, step-up, and deadlift are examples of compound exercises: They all involve flexion and extension at the ankles, knees, and hips. Isolation exercises involve movement at only one joint. Both the straight-leg hip extension (movement at the hip joint only) and the leg-curl exercise (movement at the knee joint only) are examples of lower-body isolation exercises. Compound exercises involve multiple joints and therefore multiple muscles or muscle groups. In this way, these exercises are better suited for building size and getting stronger.

Isolation exercises are best for supplementing the compound exercises and may be more appropriate for working around an injury or reconditioning an area after an injury.

EXERCISE ORDER

When you are designing your program and deciding what exercises to pair for your split, you should keep in mind that the order of the exercises is very important. Always try to do compound exercises before doing isolation exercises (especially if they involve the same muscle group). As mentioned earlier, compound exercises use multiple muscles or muscle groups and are very taxing because of this. They are often performed with much heavier loads than those for isolation exercises. You do not want to fatigue your muscles using isolation exercises before taking on the more difficult compound lifts. For example, you would not want to do isometric single-leg lifts before lunging or squatting.

Another general rule is to do free-weight exercises before machine-based movements. It takes more balance and control to lift the free weights, and you do not want to be fatigued by the machines before moving on to your free-weight exercises. However, it would be fine to do heavier machine-based compound exercises, such as the leg press, followed by free-weight seated calf raises. The isolation seated calf raise, while it is a free-weight exercise, involves only one joint (ankle) and would not be affected too much by the leg press exercise.

Using similar reasoning, try to perform your barbell exercises before dumbbell exercises. Generally you would use more weight with the barbell exercises, and you will need the extra strength to move the heavier loads of the barbell.

Finally, identify your areas of weakness and place them earlier in your workouts. This allows you to work these areas when they are most rested and get the best size and strength gains from the movements.

PART II

Lower-Body Exercises

CHAPTER 4

Gluteal Exercises

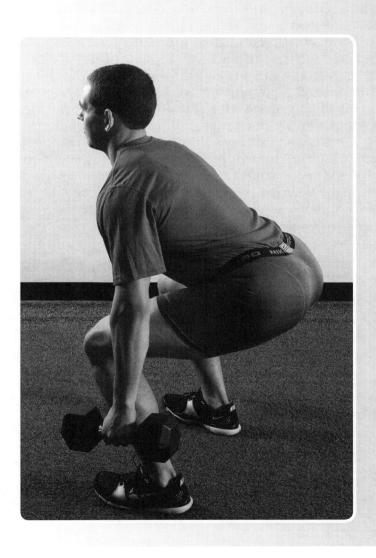

Exercises for the gluteal muscles can generally be divided into two types: compound exercises and isolation exercises. Compound exercises involve multiple joints and multiple muscle groups. The squat, for instance, is the most notable and probably the best of all glute exercises; it involves flexion and extension at the ankle, knee, and hip joints as well as recruitment of the gluteal (gluteus maximus), quadriceps (rectus femoris, vastus intermedius, vastus medialis, and vastus lateralis), and hamstring (semimembranosus, semitendinosus, and biceps femoris) muscle groups. Compound exercises are great for developing overall strength and muscle mass, so they are appropriate for a wide range of individuals.

Isolation movements involve just one joint and usually just one muscle or one muscle group. Hip-extension exercises that involve movement only at the hip joint, such as standing hip extensions, should always be done later in the workout. Both compound and isolation exercises will work the glutes; however, the quads and hamstrings are usually involved with most, if not all, compound movements and even in some of the isolation glute exercises. The lateral glute exercises, such as miniband walks and abduction machine movements, will generally work the abductor muscles (gluteus medius, gluteus minimus) as well as the adductor group (adductor brevis, adductor longus, and adductor magnus, mostly as stabilizers).

Always perform the compound exercises before the isolation exercises. The compound exercises generally involve heavier loads (and therefore develop the most strength) and require much greater effort to execute. You do not want to fatigue your legs with isolation exercises before you perform the heavier compound lifts. Doing so would compromise your strength gains and lead to possible injury.

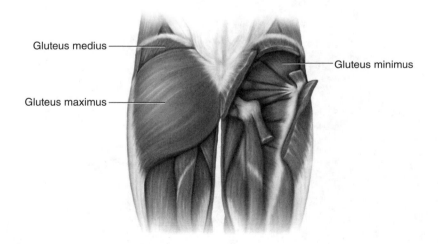

BODY-WEIGHT SQUAT

Target Glutes, quads

When Early in the workout

Start Stand with your feet just wider than shoulder-width apart. Place your hands in front of your body.

Execution Slowly descend by flexing at your hips, knees, and ankles. Lower your hips until your quads are about parallel to the floor. Keep your back straight by moving the pelvis back. Pause for one count and then return to the starting position by driving up through the middle of your feet or even through the heels of your feet. Do not hyperextend your knees at the top.

Variations Wear a weighted vest or hold a medicine ball for more resistance. An unstable surface, such as a half foam roller or DynaDisc, will add yet another progression.

Coaching Points The heels should not lift off the floor. If they do, you may be going down farther than recommended, or you may have excessive tightness in your calf and Achilles area. Focus on keeping the knees straight ahead. Hip tightness may cause the knees to collapse inward.

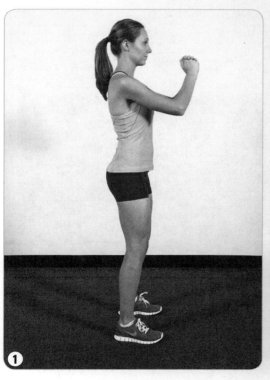

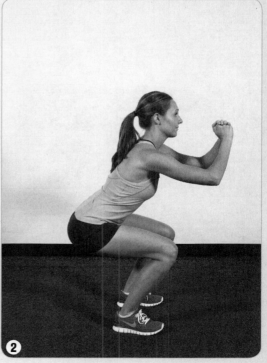

BARBELL SQUAT

Target	Glutes, quads
When	Early in the workout
Start	Place the barbell on the muscles of the upper back (not the cervical spine). Make sure your hands are equidistant from each end of the bar. Lift the bar from the rack and step back while keeping your feet about shoulder-width apart and toes turned slightly out.
Execution	Slowly descend by flexing at your hips, knees, and ankles. Lower your hips until your quads are about parallel to the floor. Keep your back straight by sticking your buttocks out. Pause for one count and then return to the starting position by driving up through the middle of your feet or even through the heels of your feet. Do not hyperextend your knees at the top.
Variations	Placing small but stable objects (many people use 5- to 10-pound plates) under your heels helps focus the movement more toward the quads. There are different types of squat bars that place the load of the bar on different parts of your upper back. Some bars put more of the load toward the posterior, which increases the gluteal involvement in the exercise.
Coaching Points	The heels should not lift off the floor. If they do, you may be going down too deep, or you may have excessive tightness in your calf and Achilles area. Focus on keeping the knees straight ahead. Hip tightness may cause the knees to collapse inward.

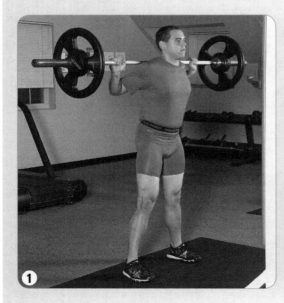

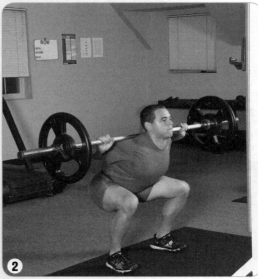

DUMBBELL SQUAT

Target	Glutes, quads
When	Early in the workout
Start	Stand with your feet just wider than shoulder-width apart. Hold a dumbbell in each hand.
Execution	Slowly descend by flexing at your hips, knees, and ankles. Lower your hips until your quads are about parallel to the floor. Keep your back straight by sticking your buttocks out. Pause for one count and then return to the starting position by driving up through the middle of your feet or even through the heels of your feet. Do not hyperextend your knees at the top.
Variations	You can also hold the dumbbells up on your shoulders to mimic a front squat. This will put a greater emphasis on your quads.
Coaching Points	The heels should not lift off the floor. If they do, you may be going down too deep, or you may have excessive tightness in your calf and Achilles area. Focus on keeping the knees straight ahead. Hip tightness may cause the knees to collapse inward.

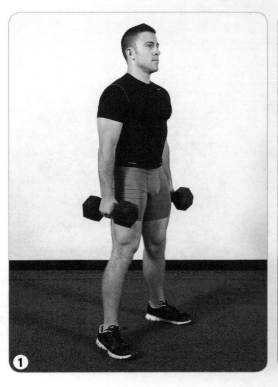

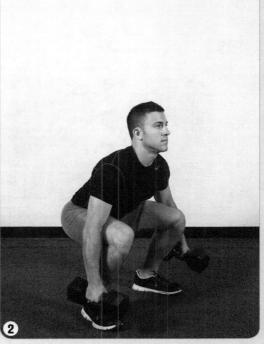

SMITH PRESS SQUAT

Target   Glutes, quads

When   Early in the workout

Start   Place the bar of the Smith press machine on the muscles of the upper back (not the cervical spine). Make sure your hands are equidistant from each end of the bar. Place your feet out in front of the midline of your body. Lift the bar from the rack and rotate the bar to release the safety hooks.

Execution   Slowly descend by flexing at your hips, knees, and ankles. Lower your hips until your quads are about parallel to the floor. Keep your back straight by sticking your buttocks out. Pause for one count and then return to the starting position by driving up through the middle of your feet or even through your heels. Do not hyperextend your knees at the top.

Variations   Changing your foot placement under the bar will functionally change the exercise. Moving your feet forward will focus more on your glutes. Be careful not to place your feet too far back underneath the bar. This foot position will not allow you to maintain proper knee flexion (knee in line with the ankle) and may result in injury.

Coaching Points Your feet should be 6 to 10 inches (15 to 25 cm) in front of your body. This will focus the exercise on the glutes. The heels should not lift off the floor. If they do, you may be going down farther than recommended, or you may have excessive tightness in your calf and Achilles area. Focus on keeping the knees straight ahead. Hip tightness may cause the knees to collapse inward.

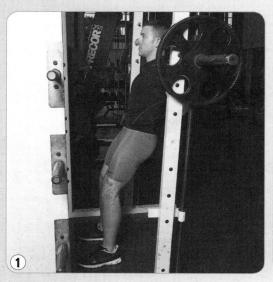
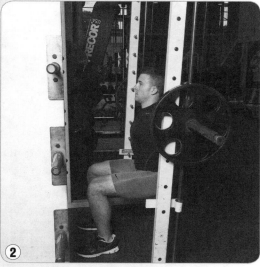

FUNCTIONAL-TRAINER SQUAT

Target	Glutes, quads
When	Early in the workout
Start	Stand with your feet just wider than shoulder-width apart. Hold the functional trainer handles in each hand at shoulder level. Keep your head up and back straight.
Execution	Slowly descend by flexing at your hips, knees, and ankles. Lower your hips until your quads are about parallel to the floor. Keep your back straight by sticking your buttocks out. Pause for one count and then return to the starting position by driving up through the middle of your feet or even through the heels of your feet. Do not hyperextend your knees at the top.
Variations	The cables will allow you to change your foot placement. Moving your feet forward will focus more on the glutes. You may also move your feet wider. A wider stance with the toes turned out will focus more on the inner thigh.
Coaching Points	Be careful not to use too much weight during this exercise. The weight is too heavy if you are unable to maintain proper posture when you are lifting the weight off the weight stack as well as when you are setting the weight back down onto the weight stack.

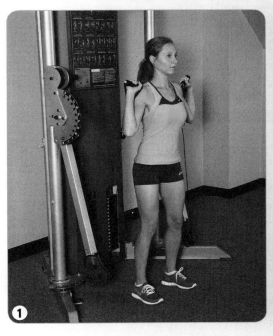 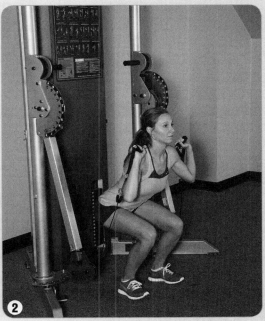

LEG PRESS

Target	Glutes, quads
When	Early in the workout
Start	Place your feet on the machine about shoulder-width apart with your feet flat and toes straight or turned slightly out. Keep your low back and midback flat against the pad and your head in a neutral position.
Execution	Extend your ankles, knees, and hips. Drive the middle portion of your feet into the platform of the machine with equal pressure from both feet. Stop the movement just short of locking your knees. Slowly return to the starting position by flexing your ankles, knees, and hips.
Variations	Adjusting the angle of the seat back will functionally change the exercise. The more you are under the machine, the greater the emphasis on the glutes. You may also change your foot placement on the platform to work the quads from different angles.
Coaching Points	Maintain contact with the back pad during the movement. Do not come off the seat. Do not go too deep into the flexed position; do maintain a flat stance on the platform with your feet.

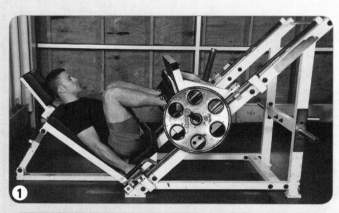

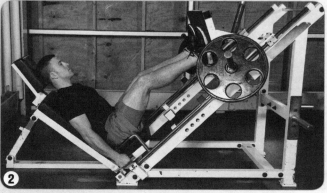

WALKING LUNGE

Target	Glutes, quads, stabilizing muscles, core
When	Early in the workout
Start	Begin standing in an upright posture with your hands together in front of your body.
Execution	Step forward with one foot and flex your ankle, knee, and hip until your lead foot is flat on the floor with your knee at a 90-degree angle. Your back leg should be flexed, the knee just short of touching the floor. Drive forward by extending your ankle, knee, and hip with the ball of the foot of the lead leg and the toes of the back leg. Repeat this movement with the opposite leg, and continue alternating sides in a walking manner.
Variations	Hold a medicine ball, weight plate, or dumbbell in both hands for greater resistance. The extra weight also calls upon the core muscles to provide stabilization during the exercise.
Coaching Points	Step far enough out in front so that the knee stays over the ankle and does not go out over the toes. Keep the torso in an upright posture.

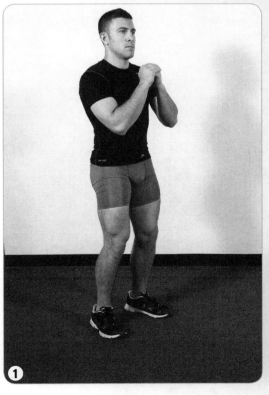

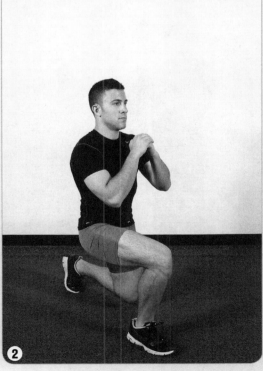

WALKING LUNGE WITH ROTATION

Target	Glutes, quads, stabilizing muscles, core
When	Early in the workout
Start	Begin by standing in an upright posture with your hands together and in front of your body.
Execution	Step forward with one foot and flex your ankle, knee, and hip. At the same time, rotate your upper body in the direction of the lead leg until your lead foot is flat on the floor with your knee at a 90-degree angle. Your back leg should be flexed, and the knee just short of touching the floor. Drive forward by extending your ankle, knee, and hip with the ball of the foot of the lead leg and the toes of the back leg. Rotate the torso back to the neutral position, facing forward. Repeat this movement with the opposite leg, and continue alternating sides in a walking manner.
Variations	Hold a medicine ball, weight plate, or dumbbell in both hands during the rotation for greater resistance. The extra weight also calls upon the core muscles to provide stabilization during the exercise.
Coaching Points	Step far enough out in front of you so that the knee stays over the ankle and does not go out over the toes. Keep the torso in an upright posture.

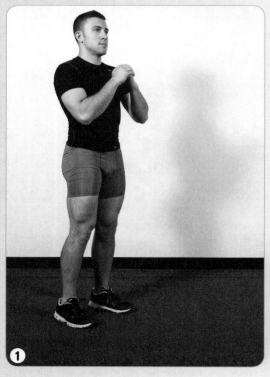

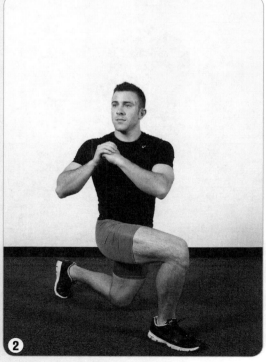

BENCH SINGLE-LEG SQUAT

Target Glutes, quads

When Early in the workout

Start Place the top of one foot on a bench or stable step that is approximately 22 to 24 inches (55 to 60 cm) high. Place the opposite leg out in front of you with your knee slightly bent and your foot flat on the floor. Keep your hands out in front of your body while maintaining an upright posture with your upper body.

Execution Descend straight down with your upper body by flexing the ankle and knee of your forward leg. Once your knee flexes to 90 degrees, stop the descent and return back up to the start position by driving up through the heel of your foot and extending your knee.

Variations Some people find it more comfortable to do this exercise with the ball of the foot of the nonworking leg on the bench. Holding dumbbells or wearing a weighted vest adds greater resistance. Placing the resting leg on an exercise ball also increases the intensity.

Coaching Points Do not let the knee of the working (forward) leg go out over the toes. Keep an upright posture with a wide stance to alleviate this problem.

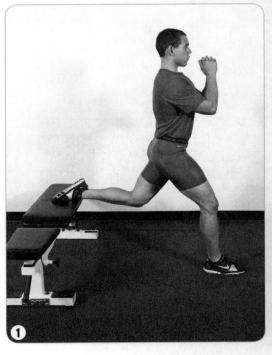
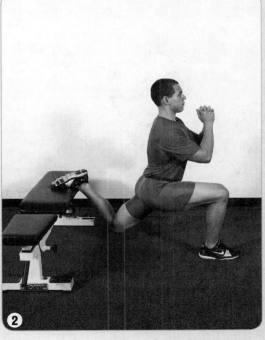

STEP-UP

Target	Glutes, quads
When	Early to middle of the workout
Start	Place one foot flat and entirely on a bench or box that is 12 to 18 inches (30 to 46 cm) high. Keep your back flat and your head in a neutral position. Place your hands together directly in front of you.
Execution	Drive up through the heel of the foot that is on the box or bench by extending your knee and hip. Raise the nondriving leg up until the knee is flexed at 90 degrees. Return the nondriving leg slowly to the floor and lightly touch the ball of your foot before beginning your next repetition.
Variations	Varying the height of the box adds variety and changes the focus from glutes (higher) to quads (lower). Stepping up from the side of the box works your lateral rotators and adductors as well.
Coaching Points	Tempo is the key to this exercise. Use the momentum of the nondriving leg rather than the driving leg and return to the start slowly. Sit back and focus on extending your hip with your glutes. Do not let your knee get out over your toes.

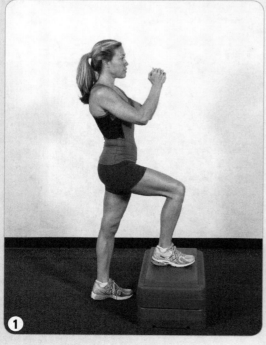
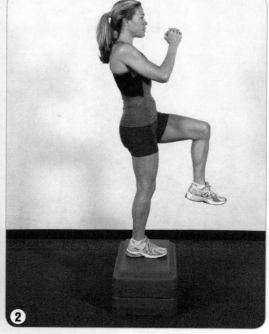

STEP-DOWN

Target Glutes, quads

When Middle of the workout

Start Stand with one foot entirely on, but slightly to the side of, a box or step that is 6 to 12 inches (15 to 30 cm) high. Extend the opposite leg slightly out in front of the body. Keep the foot dorsiflexed.

Execution Slowly flex the ankle, knee, and hip of the leg that is on the box until the heel of your extended foot lightly touches the floor. Return to the starting position by driving up through the heel of the foot that is on the box and extending that ankle, knee, and hip.

Variations Reach out in front of your body with the nonworking leg for greater glute involvement of the working leg.

Coaching Points Keep your weight back toward your heel and do not let the knee of the working leg drift out over the toes. You may want to stand near a wall and lightly touch it for stability if needed.

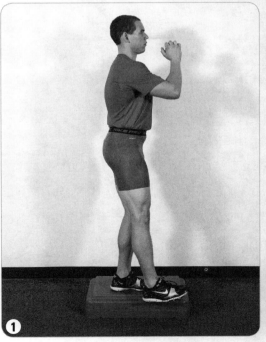 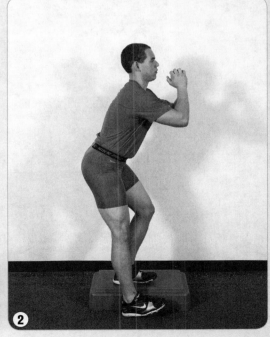

SINGLE-LEG PRESS

Target	Glutes, quads
When	Middle of the workout
Start	Place one foot on the machine with your foot flat and toes straight or turned slightly out. Keep your low back and midback flat against the pad and your head in a neutral position.
Execution	Extend your ankle, knee, and hip. Drive the middle portion of your foot into the platform of the machine. Stop the movement just short of locking your knee. Slowly return to the starting position by flexing your ankle, knee, and hip.
Variations	Adjusting the angle of the seat back will functionally change the exercise. The more you are under the machine, the greater the emphasis is on the glutes. You may also change your foot placement on the platform to work the quads from different angles.
Coaching Points	Maintain contact with the back pad during the movement. Do not come off the seat. Do not go too deep into the flexed position; do maintain a flat stance on the platform with your foot.

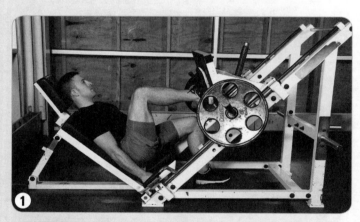

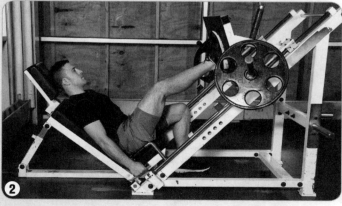

4-WAY HIP-MACHINE EXTENSION

Target	Glutes, hamstrings
When	Middle of the workout
Start	Place one leg on top of the pad just under your knee. Keep the opposite foot flat on the platform with your toe pointing straight ahead and the knee slightly bent. Stand tall with your upper body and hold onto the support rails of the machine.
Execution	Push down on the pad of the machine by extending your hip and knee. Go slightly past the midline of your body. Return to the start position slowly by resisting the weight of the stack.
Variations	To focus more on the glutes and minimize hamstring involvement, place the arm of the machine in a lower position and perform the movement with a straight leg.
Coaching Points	Make sure the axis of the machine is in line with your hip. Do not hyperextend your back at the end of the downward phase of the movement.

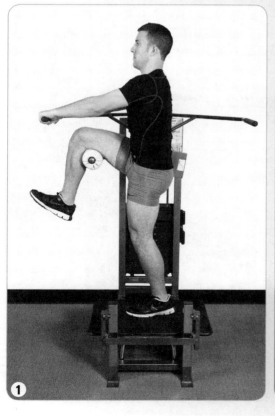
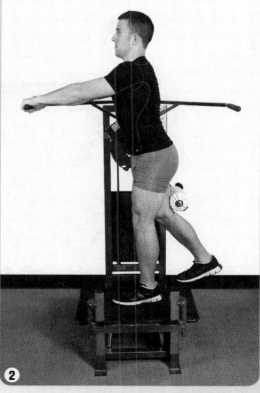

ANKLE-WEIGHT STANDING HIP EXTENSION

Target	Glutes, hamstrings
When	Late in the workout
Start	Wrap 5- to 25-pound ankle weights around your ankle. Stand on a 4- to 6-inch step (10 to 15 cm) with the nonweighted foot, keeping a slight bend in this knee. Stand in an upright posture while holding onto a wall or secure object.
Execution	Slowly extend the working hip until your foot is about 12 to 24 inches (30 to 60 cm) behind you. Return slowly until your weighted foot is in line with the support leg.
Variations	Try leaning over a training table or other object that will support your upper body. The table should be around hip height. This prevents you from swaying your upper body.
Coaching Points	Do not extend your leg behind you to the extent that you hyperextend your low back.

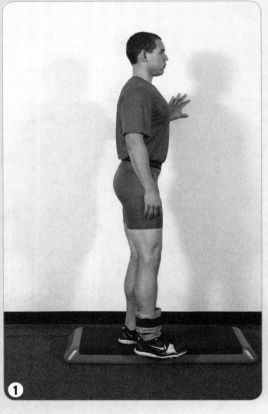 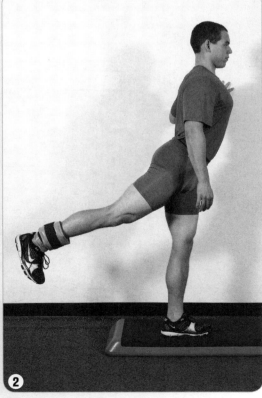

ANKLE-WEIGHT ALL-FOURS HIP EXTENSION

Target	Glutes, hamstrings
When	Late in the workout
Start	Wrap 5- to 25-pound ankle weights around your ankles. Get into an all-fours stance with your head up and back straight.
Execution	Extend one leg back until it is almost straight. Slowly return to the start position, keeping your knee off the floor.
Variations	A variation of this exercise that targets the upper glutes and outer hips is to abduct your hip and then extend your leg straight back.
Coaching Points	Do not hyperextend your back by going too fast and reaching too high with your foot.

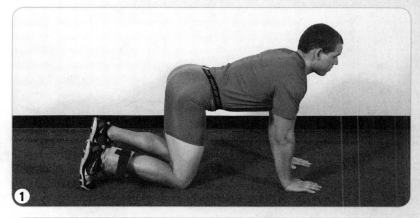

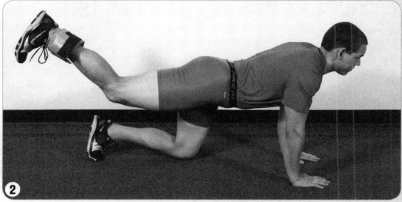

MINIBAND HIP EXTENSION

Target   Glutes, hamstrings

When   Late in the workout

Start   Place the resistance-band loop (miniband) around both ankles. Stand in an upright posture facing a wall with both arms extended and hands against the wall. Keep a slight bend in the knee of the support leg.

Execution   Slowly extend your hip until your foot is about 12 to 24 inches (30 to 60 cm) behind you. Return slowly until your working foot is in line with the support leg.

Variations   There are many levels of resistance bands. Try heavier bands for greater resistance. You may also try placing a second band just above your knees.

Coaching Points   Do not extend your leg behind you to the extent that you hyper-extend your low back.

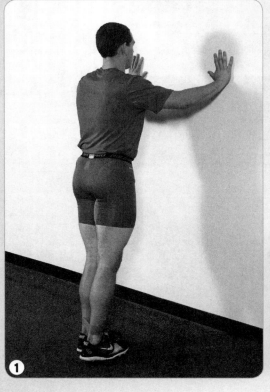
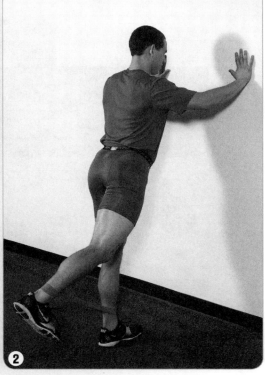

EXERCISE-BALL LYING HIP EXTENSION

Target   Glutes, low back

When   Late in the workout

Start   Place an exercise ball under your waist with your arms straight and in a push-up position. Keep your legs straight and feet a few inches apart with your toes pointing down and resting on the floor. Keep your head in a neutral position.

Execution   Raise your feet off the floor by extending your hips. Keep your knees locked throughout the entire movement. Return to the starting position.

Variations   Place the ball on a sturdy table or bench and perform the exercise. This gives you a much greater range of motion.

Coaching Points Keep your upper body still and do not collapse your arms. Extend your hips until your legs are in a straight line with the rest of your body. Do not hyperextend your back. Keep your toes pointed down throughout the movement.

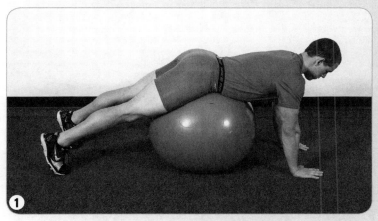

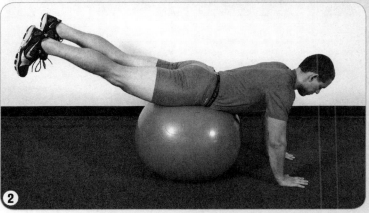

DOUBLE-LEG BRIDGE

Target	Glutes, hamstrings
When	Late in the workout
Start	Lie on your back with your knees bent and arms at your sides. Keep your feet flat on the floor. Your heels should be approximately 12 inches (30 cm) from your buttocks.
Execution	Raise your hips off the floor by contracting your glutes and hamstrings and driving your heels into the floor. Stop the movement once your spine is in a neutral position. Return slowly to the start position.
Variations	You can perform this movement with only your heels on the floor rather than with feet flat. You can also try this with your feet or heels on an exercise ball or medicine ball.
Coaching Points	Do not push into the floor with your head, neck, or arms. Stop the movement as soon as your spine is in a neutral position. Do not hyperextend your back.

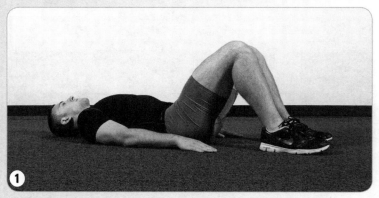

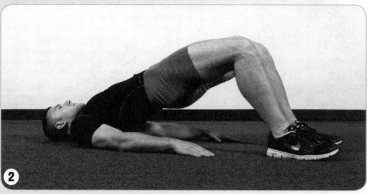

SINGLE-LEG BRIDGE

Target	Glutes, hamstrings
When	Late in the workout
Start	Lie on your back with your knees bent and arms at your sides. Keep one foot flat on the floor. Your heel should be approximately 12 inches (30 cm) from your buttocks. Raise your opposite foot off the floor and flex the knee to 90 degrees. Hold the flexed leg in the 90-degree position during the movement.
Execution	Raise your hips off the floor by contracting your glutes and hamstrings and driving your heel into the floor. Stop the movement once your spine is in a neutral position. Return slowly to the start position.
Variations	You can perform this movement with only your heel on the floor rather than a flat foot; this creates instability and adds intensity to the exercise.
Coaching Points	Do not push into the floor with your head, neck, or arms. Make sure you keep your hips level throughout the movement. Stop the movement as soon as your spine is in a neutral position. Do not hyperextend your back.

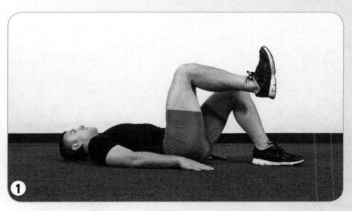

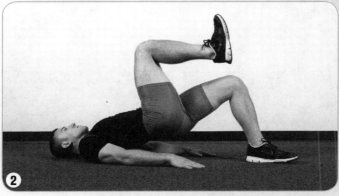

MINIBAND LATERAL WALK

Target	Glutes (lateral rotators)
When	Late in the workout
Start	Place the resistance-band loop (miniband) around both ankles. Stand in an upright posture with both feet pointing straight ahead and your hands on your hips.
Execution	Step laterally about 12 to 18 inches (30 to 46 cm) with the lead leg. Keep your feet and toes pointing straight forward. Step with the trailing leg about half of the distance of the lead leg (6 to 9 inches or 15 to 23 cm). Keep both legs straight during each step.
Variations	For greater resistance you can place another band around your legs just above your knees.
Coaching Points	Do not drag your feet. Take deliberate steps and do not sway your upper body. Your trunk should stay in a straight line the entire time.

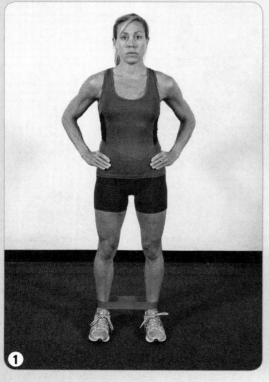
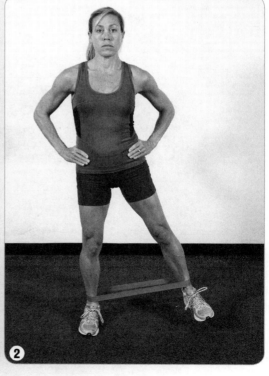

ROMAN CHAIR REVERSE HYPEREXTENSION

Target   Glutes, hamstrings, low back

When   Late in the workout

Start   Begin with your hips on the pads of the Roman chair. Hold onto the platform, where your feet would normally go, with both hands. Keep your head in a neutral position.

Execution   Raise both legs up until they are in line with your spine. Hold for one count and then return slowly to the starting position.

Variations   For greater resistance, you can hold a medicine ball or dumbbell between your feet.

Coaching Points Make sure you move slowly in both directions of the lift. Avoid using momentum and do not hyperextend your back.

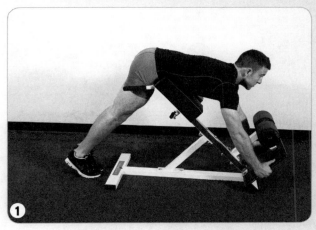

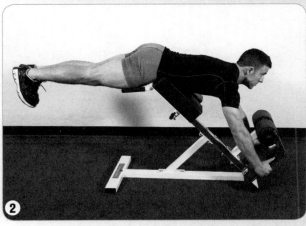

SLED PUSH

Target	Glutes, quads, hamstrings, low back
When	Late in the workout
Start	Hold the sled with your head up and spine in a neutral position. Stagger your feet so that one foot is in front of the other. Begin on the balls of both feet.
Execution	Push off of the floor with the rear foot and drive your knees toward your chest, alternating feet in a good running form. Proceed in this manner for the prescribed number of reps or distance.
Variations	For greater resistance, you can add weight to the sled. This will work the muscles at a greater intensity. Walking and pushing the sled is a good way to learn the exercise and then progress to running.
Coaching Points	Keep your head up and your neck and spine in a neutral position.

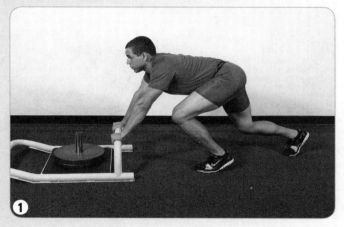

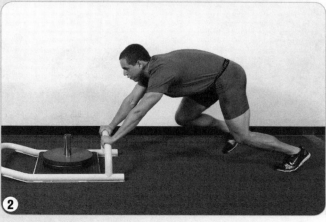

FUNCTIONAL-TRAINER HIP EXTENSION

Target	Glutes, hamstrings
When	End of the workout
Start	Set the arm of the functional trainer to its lowest position. Secure the strap tightly around your ankle with the clasp facing the machine. Stand on a 4- to 6-inch step (10 to 15 cm) with the opposite foot. Keep a slight bend in this knee. Stand in an upright posture while holding onto the machine for balance.
Execution	Slowly extend your hip until your foot is about 12 to 24 inches (30 to 60 cm) behind you. Return slowly until your involved foot is in line with the support leg.
Variations	Slightly rotating your hip inward or outward works the glutes from a slightly different angle.
Coaching Points	Do not extend your leg so far behind you that you hyperextend your low back.

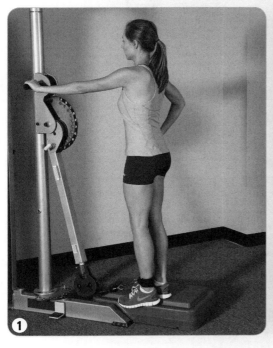 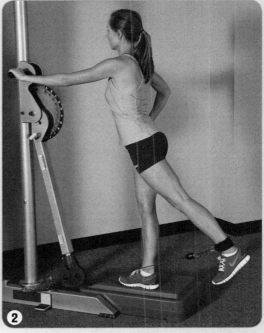

RESISTANCE-BAND HIP EXTENSION

Target	Glutes, hamstrings
When	End of the workout
Start	Lie on your back with a strap securely around your foot or ankle. Attach the resistance band to the front of the strap on the top of the working foot or ankle. Secure the band to a sturdy object above your head and about 5 feet (1.5 m) off the floor. Your head should be facing in the direction of the resistance-band attachment. Keep the opposite leg bent with your foot flat on the floor.
Execution	Begin the movement with your leg straight and hip flexed at a 90-degree angle. Extend your leg down toward the floor. Slowly return to the start position while resisting the tubing.
Variations	Add a second resistance band to make the exercise more demanding.
Coaching Points	Keep your low back against the floor and relax your head and neck.

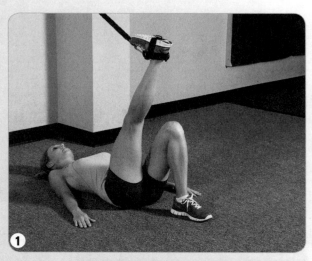

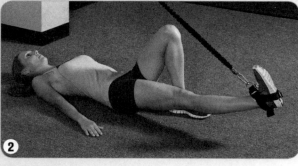

CHAPTER 5

Quadriceps Exercises

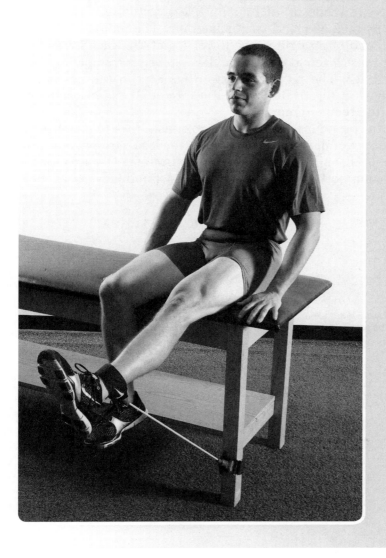

The quadriceps, or quads, make up the upper portion of the medial front side, the middle, and the lateral side of the legs. The quad muscles are used for supporting the body in a standing position. Because the major leg muscles are close together and work together to perform various movements, compound exercises that use multiple joints and multiple muscles make up a large number of quad exercises. Exercises such as in-place lunges and front squats involve the quads and glutes as well as other stabilizing and supportive musculature and are great compound exercises for developing size and strength in the thighs. The leg-extension machine is probably the best example of an isolation quad exercise (an exercise involving a single joint or single muscle or muscle group). There is very little stabilizing muscle activation during this exercise.

The quadriceps are made up of four muscles: rectus femoris, vastus intermedius, vastus medialis, and vastus lateralis. The main function of the quads is to extend or straighten the lower leg at the knee joint. This is the reason that most lifters consider the leg extension a staple exercise in their quad routines. The rectus femoris originates in the pelvis and therefore is involved in hip flexion as well. Compound exercises are the best way to train the rectus femoris.

Maximizing both compound and isolation exercises for the quads is the best way to increase overall size and strength in the legs. Strong and stable quads enhance athletic ability, make it easier to perform the activities of everyday life, help support the knee joint, and assist in injury prevention.

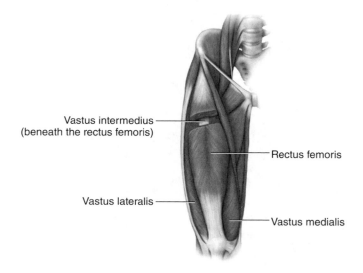

Vastus intermedius (beneath the rectus femoris)

Rectus femoris

Vastus lateralis

Vastus medialis

BARBELL SQUAT ON WEIGHT PLATES

Target	Quads, glutes
When	Early in the workout
Start	Place the barbell across the muscular portion of your upper back so that the bulk of the weight lies across the traps, not on the cervical vertebrae. Begin with your feet just wider than shoulder-width apart. Carefully step onto 5- or 10-pound flat weight plates with your heels, keeping the front part of your feet on the floor.
Execution	Lower your body by flexing at your ankles, knees, and hips. Descend until your quads are about parallel to the floor. Return to the start position by extending the ankles, knees, and hips.
Variations	You can also use dumbbells for this exercise. Place a dumbbell in each hand; then flex your elbows and hold the dumbbells on your deltoids. You can also hold dumbbells at your side for added resistance.
Coaching Points	Make sure your weight plates (or any other object that you might use) are not slippery or unstable.

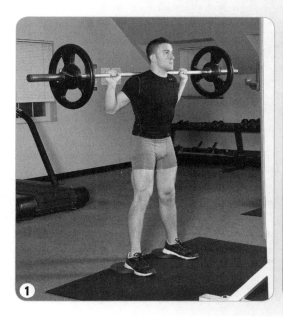

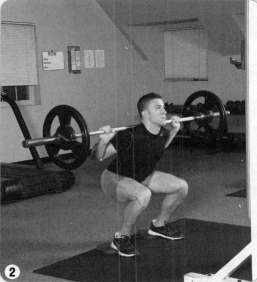

FRONT SQUAT

Target	Quads, glutes
When	Early in the workout
Start	Place your feet just wider than shoulder-width apart. Place the barbell across the middle portion of your deltoids. Hold the bar with a pronated grip and just outside of your shoulders.
Execution	Lower your body by flexing at your ankles, knees, and hips. Descend until your quads are about parallel to the floor. Return to the start position by extending the ankles, knees, and hips.
Variations	You can also use dumbbells for this exercise. Place a dumbbell in each hand, and then flex your elbows and hold the dumbbells on your deltoids. This neutral grip position allows those who have poor wrist flexibility to perform the front squat without discomfort.
Coaching Points	Be very careful with the placement of the bar or dumbbells on your shoulder area. The barbell may be difficult to balance, so start with a light weight until you master the movement. People with wrist tightness or injury may have difficultly holding the bar in this position.

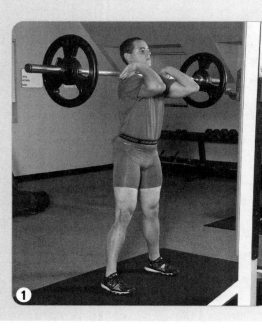
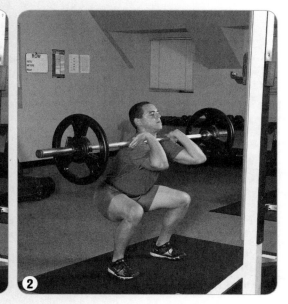

EXERCISE-BALL SQUAT

Target	Quads, glutes
When	Early in the workout
Start	Stand about 2 to 3 feet (1 to 2 m) away from a solid wall with your feet slightly wider than shoulder-width apart. Place an exercise ball between the wall and your low back. Keep pressure on the ball by slightly leaning back against it.
Execution	Slowly descend by flexing at your hips, knees, and ankles. Lower your body until your quads are approximately parallel to the floor. Keep your back straight and look straight ahead. Pause for one count and then return to the starting position by driving up through the heels of your feet. Do not lock out your knees at the top.
Variations	You may hold dumbbells or wear a weighted vest during this exercise to add resistance.
Coaching Points	Make sure the exercise ball is placed properly in the small of your low back. Your knees should be well behind your toes when in the flexed position.

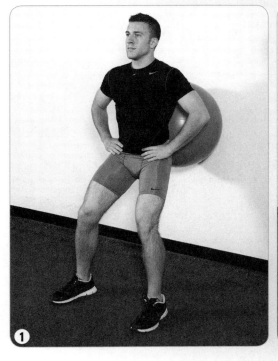
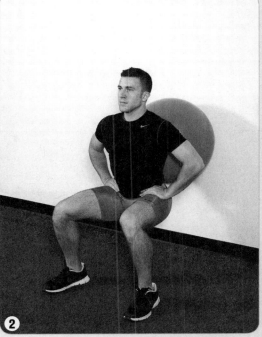

SPLIT SQUAT

Target	Quads, glutes, hamstrings
When	Early in the workout
Start	Place your feet in a split position with one foot out in front of you and one foot behind you. Bend your front leg so that the knee forms a 90-degree angle. Move your rear leg if necessary to accommodate the angle. The back leg should be bent and your body weight evenly dispersed between the front foot and back foot. Keep your torso upright with hands in front of your body.
Execution	Slowly descend until your back knee lightly touches the floor. Do not bounce or rest on the floor with the back knee. Drive up through the heel of the front foot and the ball of the back foot. Extend upward until your knees are almost straight.
Variations	This exercise can be made more challenging by wearing a weighted vest, holding a medicine ball, or holding a dumbbell in each hand to further challenge the muscles. An unstable surface under the front foot also challenges the muscles to maintain balance and stability.
Coaching Points	You may have a tendency to lunge forward during this exercise. Make sure your torso is upright and that the front knee stays in line with the front ankle. Do not lean forward or let the knee go out over the toes. Keep toes pointing straight ahead.

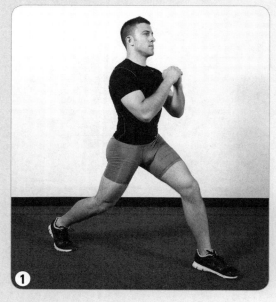
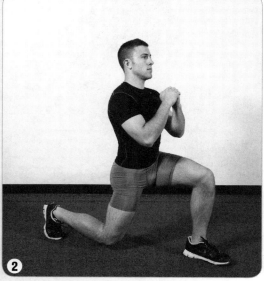

SINGLE-LEG SQUAT

Target	Quads, glutes, hamstrings
When	Early in the workout
Start	Stand on one foot about 16 inches (40 cm) away from a 6- to 12-inch cone (15 to 30 cm). Extend your hands out in front of you. Keep your opposite leg flexed and slightly behind the midline of your body.
Execution	Flex the knee and hip of the working leg and squat down toward the cone. Reach toward the cone with both arms extended. Lightly touch the cone and then extend your knee and hip by driving up through the heel of your foot. Your nonworking leg will extend behind you with a slight bend at the knee.
Variations	Place cones in a half circle out in front of you and reach with your opposite hand across your body to touch each cone as you squat. This changes your center of gravity and forces the muscles to work harder to stabilize the lower body.
Coaching Points	Make sure you sit back during the squat movement. You do not want the knee of the involved leg going out over your toes. Keep your head up and back straight. Do not bend too far forward at the hips.

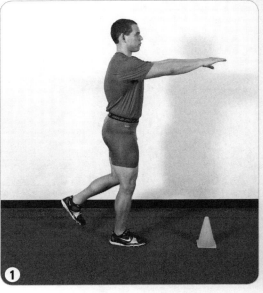

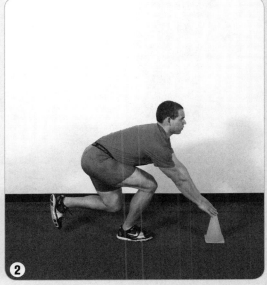

IN-PLACE LUNGE

Target   Quads, glutes, hamstrings

When   Early in the workout

Start   Begin standing in an upright posture with your hands on your hips.

Execution   Step forward with one foot and flex your ankle, knee, and hip until your lead foot is flat on the floor with your knee at a 90-degree angle. Your back knee should be flexed and just short of touching the floor. Drive backward by extending the ankle, knee, and hip of the lead leg to return to the starting position. Repeat this movement with the opposite leg.

Variations   Add a weighted vest, medicine ball, or dumbbells to this exercise for greater resistance.

Coaching Points Step far enough out in front so that the knee stays over the ankle and does not go out over the toes. Keep the torso in an upright posture.

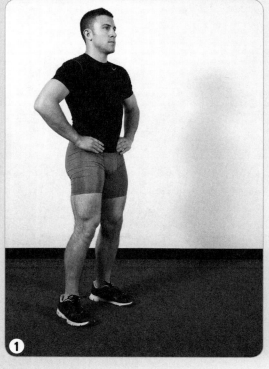

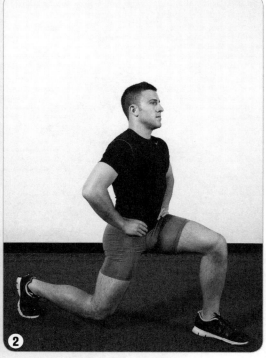

WEIGHTED-SLED WALKING LUNGE

Target Quads, glutes, hamstrings

When Early in the workout

Start Begin by standing in an upright position with your hands on your hips and the weighted sled secured tightly around your waist with an appropriate harness.

Execution Step forward with one foot and flex your ankle, knee, and hip until your lead foot is flat on the floor with your knee at a 90-degree angle. Your back leg should be flexed and just short of touching the floor. Drive forward by extending your ankle, knee, and hip, pushing off with the ball of the foot of the lead leg and the toes of the back leg. Continue this movement with the opposite leg in a walking manner.

Variations You can add upper body rotation to this movement for extra core work and muscle stabilization.

Coaching Points Step far enough in front of you that the knee stays over the ankle and does not go out over the toes. Keep the torso in an upright position. Make sure your strap is sturdy and long enough that it does not slide into your back leg or foot.

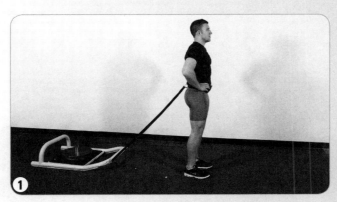

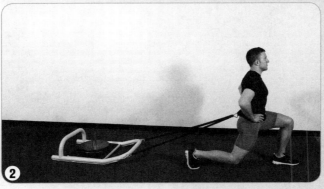

WALKING RETRO LUNGE

Target Quads, glutes, hamstrings

When Early in the workout

Start Begin standing in an upright position with your hands on your hips.

Execution Step back with one foot by extending your hip and flexing your knee until the ball of your foot is on the floor. Your front leg should be flexed, with your knee at 90 degrees and the foot flat on the floor. Drive backward by extending your front knee and hip until you are back to the start position. Repeat this movement with the opposite leg in a backward-walking motion.

Variations This exercise can be performed in place, but it changes the dynamic of the exercise, focusing slightly more on the glutes.

Coaching Points Step back far enough that your front knee is at 90 degrees and your knee is in line with your ankle.

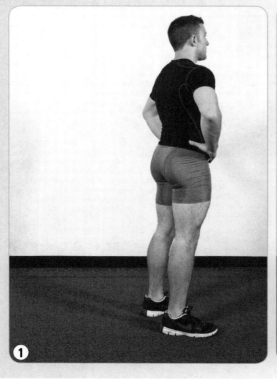
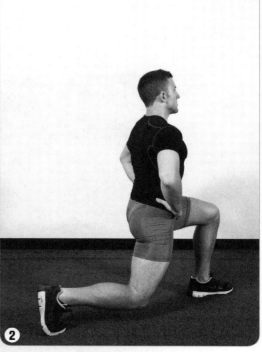

DROP LUNGE

Target	Quads, glutes, hamstrings
When	Early in the workout
Start	Begin standing in an upright position with your hands on your hips.
Execution	Step back and across the midline of your body with one foot by extending that hip and flexing your knee until the ball of your foot is on the floor. Your front leg should be flexed with the knee bent at 90 degrees and the foot flat on the floor. Drive back up by extending your front knee and hip until you are back to the start position. Repeat this movement with the opposite leg.
Variations	This exercise can be performed by alternating the legs. It will not change the effect on the muscles, but it will challenge your sense of balance and your cardiovascular system.
Coaching Points	Step back and across your body's midline (crossing over your opposite leg). Step far enough back that your front knee is at 90 degrees and in line with your ankle.

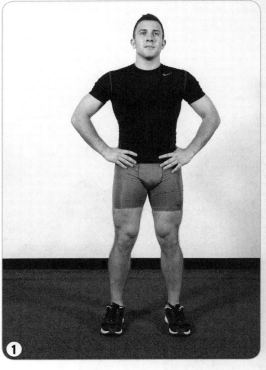

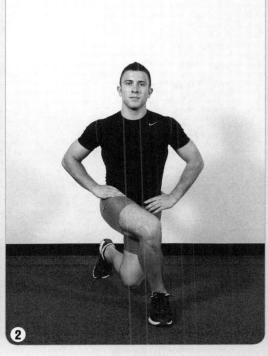

LATERAL LUNGE

Target	Quads, glutes, hamstrings, adductors
When	Early in the workout
Start	Stand with your arms relaxed and at your sides. Keep both feet about 6 inches (15 cm) apart.
Execution	Slowly flex your hip and knee of one leg until the knee is just below 90 degrees and your foot is off of the floor. Step laterally about 3 or 4 feet (1 m) with this same leg and land softly on your foot. Straddle your opposite knee with each arm while keeping your head up and back straight. Sit back with the majority of your weight on the stationary leg. Keep your toes pointed straight ahead and both feet flat on the floor. Drive off the laterally extended leg and return to the start position.
Variations	Add resistance by holding dumbbells, weighted bar, or medicine ball.
Coaching Points	Make sure you do not overstride on your lateral step. Work your way out slowly through trial and error. Keep your weight back and toward your heels; this will help you keep your knees in line with your ankles.

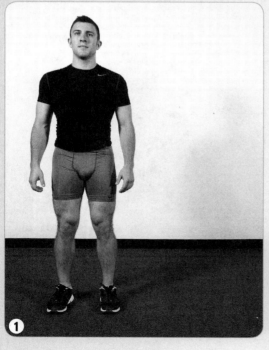
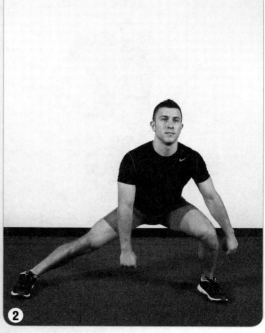

SLIDE LATERAL LUNGE

Target	Quads, glutes, hamstrings, adductors, abductors
When	Early to middle of the workout
Start	Stand with your arms relaxed and at your sides. Keep your feet about 6 inches (15 cm) apart. Place the slide under the ball of the foot that will move laterally. Keep most of your body weight on the stable leg.
Execution	Flex the hip and knee of the stationary leg while very slowly sliding your opposite leg out to the side. Straddle your stationary knee with each arm. Slide your moving leg to a comfortable position. Drive up through the foot of the stationary leg while keeping your head up and back straight. Return to the starting position.
Variations	Hold a dumbbell in each hand for greater resistance.
Coaching Points	Make sure your first repetition does not slide out too far from your stationary leg. Gradually increase the distance as you become more comfortable but be very careful not to overextend your slide leg.

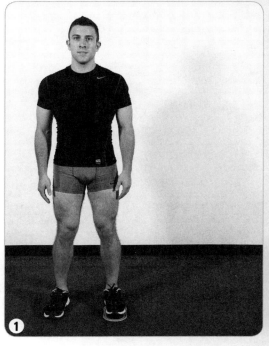

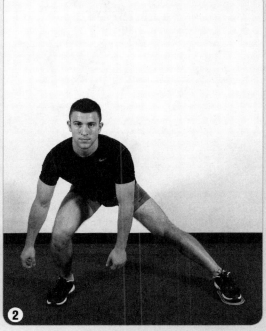

BODY-WEIGHT WIDE SQUAT

Target	Quads, glutes, adductors
When	Middle of the workout
Start	Stand with your feet about 6 to 8 inches (15 to 20 cm) wider than shoulder-width apart. Turn your feet out to the side at about a 45-degree angle. Place your hands in front of your body.
Execution	Slowly descend by flexing your hips, knees, and ankles. Lower your hips until your quads are approximately parallel to the floor. Keep your knees in line with your toes as you descend. Drive up through the middle of your feet as you return to the starting position. Do not lock your knees at the top.
Variations	Hold a weighted plate, a dumbbell, or medicine ball, or wear a weighted vest for added resistance.
Coaching Points	Most people feel tightness in the groin area during the descending movement. Try to keep your knees from collapsing inward due to this tightness. Working through this tightness helps increase your range of motion throughout the hip region.

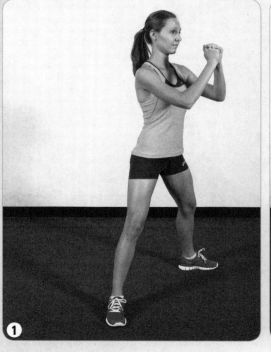
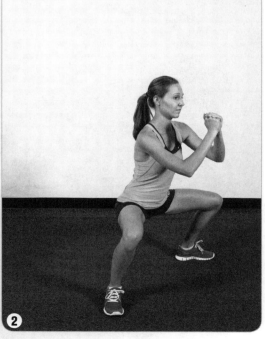

STRAIGHT-LEG STEP-DOWN

Target	Quads, glutes, hamstrings
When	Middle of the workout
Start	Stand with one foot entirely on but slightly to the side of a box or step that is 6 to12 inches (15 to 30 cm) high. Keep the opposite leg straight down and to the side of the box.
Execution	Slowly flex the ankle, knee, and hip of the leg that is on the box until the heel of your extended foot lightly touches the floor. Return to the starting position by driving up through the middle or front of the foot of the working leg and extending that ankle, knee, and hip.
Variations	Use a bench or higher step to increase the intensity.
Coaching Points	If necessary, stand near a wall so that you can lightly touch it to stabilize yourself.

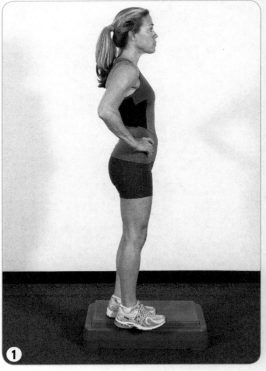
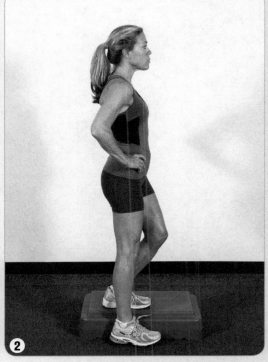

BENCH SINGLE-LEG SIT

Target	Quads, glutes, hamstrings
When	Middle of the workout
Start	Stand on one leg about 6 to 8 inches (15 to 20 cm) in front of a stable exercise bench. Bend the opposite leg at the knee and keep this leg slightly out in front of your body.
Execution	Slowly sit down onto the bench by flexing your ankle, knee, and hip of the involved leg. Keep the opposite leg flexed and out in front of your body. Sit on the bench for one count and then drive back up to the starting position. Repeat with the opposite leg.
Variations	Beginners may perform the first part of the exercise (the sitting portion) with both legs and then stand with a single leg. This will take away some of the intensity of the exercise while continuing to work the muscles the same way.
Coaching Points	The eccentric (lowering) part of the exercise is key to this movement. Go slowly and with control on the way down to the bench. Do not drop onto the bench. Drive back up by pushing through the heel of the foot that is on the floor. Maintain proper posture by keeping your head, neck, and spine in a neutral position.

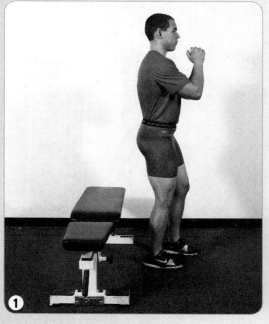 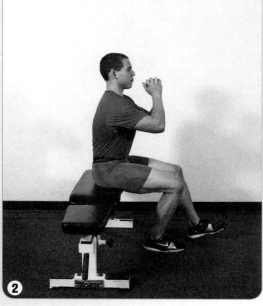

MACHINE LEG EXTENSION

Target	Quads
When	Middle to end of the workout
Start	Adjust the back of the seat so that the axis of the machine is in line with your knees. Adjust the shin pad so that it is just above your ankles. Sit up straight with your back against the pad. Point your toes up.
Execution	Extend both legs slowly until the knees are just short of being locked. Return to the starting position in a slow, controlled manner.
Variations	Turning your feet slightly out (targeting the vastus medialis) or slightly in (targeting the vastus lateralis) will work the quads in a functionally different way. Try this exercise while holding a soccer ball between your knees to put extra emphasis on the vastus medialis.
Coaching Points	Make sure you do not round your low spine. Sit up tall. If you have a history of knee pain, limit your range of motion in the flexion phase of this exercise.

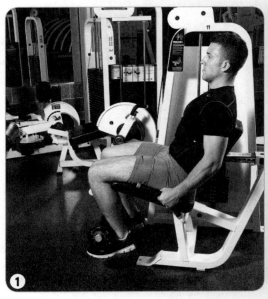 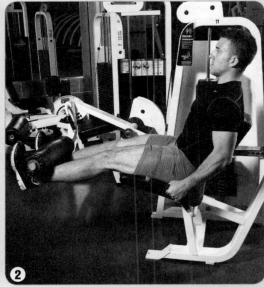

MINIBAND LOW LATERAL WALK

Target   Quads, glutes, abductors

When   Late in the workout

Start   Place the resistance band (miniband) around both ankles. Stand on the balls of your feet with your knees flexed. Place your hands on your hips. Keep your head up and your back straight.

Execution   Step laterally about 12 to 18 inches (30 to 46 cm) with the lead leg. Keep your feet and toes pointing straight ahead. Step with the trailing leg about half of the distance of the lead leg (6 to 9 inches or 15 to 22 cm). Keep both legs flexed and stay on the balls of your feet during each step.

Variations   Hold a medicine ball or weighted plate while performing this exercise for added resistance.

Coaching Points Do not drag your feet. Take deliberate steps and do not sway your upper body. Your trunk should stay in a straight line the entire time. You may have a tendency to stand up during the movement. Keep the knees flexed throughout the exercise.

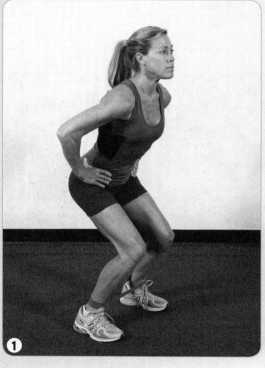
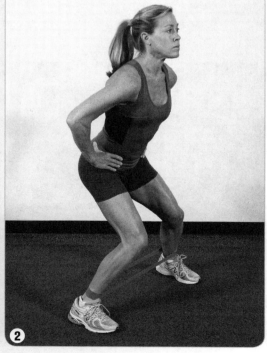

FUNCTIONAL-TRAINER LEG EXTENSION

Target	Quads
When	Late in the workout
Start	Sit on a stable training table or bench. Secure an ankle strap with a hook around your ankle and attach the hook to the functional trainer. Sit up straight with your hands at your sides. Point your toes up.
Execution	Extend your leg until it is almost straight but not locked. Return slowly to the start position.
Variations	You can perform this exercise while standing if there is no table or bench available. Flex your leg at the hip and point your toes up. Extend your knee. This method is much more difficult, and you should use much less weight than when seated. Standing also challenges the muscles of the nonworking leg to maintain balance and stability.
Coaching Points	Do not flex your knee greater than 90 degrees during the downward phase of the movement.

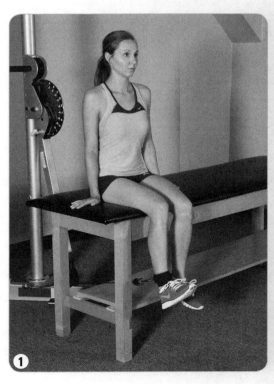 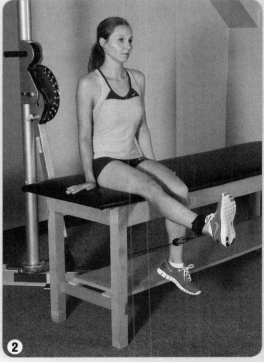

FUNCTIONAL-TRAINER STRAIGHT-LEG HIP FLEXION

Target   Quads, hip flexors

When   Late in the workout

Start   Secure the strap of the cable around your ankle. Face away from the machine while standing on a 6-inch step (15 cm) with your opposite foot.

Execution   Extend your leg at the hip while keeping your knee locked. Return slowly to the start position.

Variations   This exercise can also be performed using resistance bands or ankle weights if a functional trainer is not available.

Coaching Points   This is an excellent isometric quad exercise for those who may have knee discomfort.

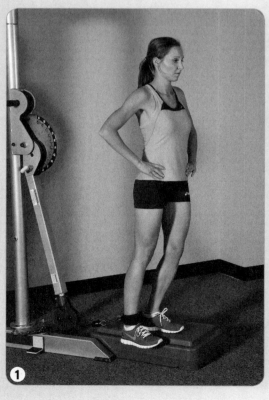
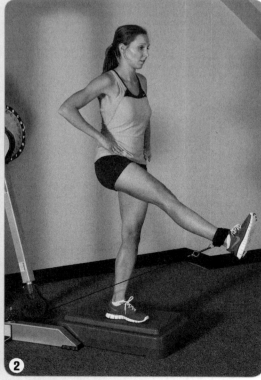

MANUAL-RESISTANCE LEG EXTENSION

Target	Quads
When	Late in the workout
Start	Sit on the end of a training table or other object that is high enough so that your feet are off the floor. Make sure the edge of the table is right behind the knee joints. A trainer or training partner should place one hand just above the ankle joint.
Execution	Extend your leg until it is almost straight but not locked. Resist the pressure of the trainer's hand on the up and down phase. Stop at 90 degrees of knee flexion on the downward phase.
Variations	The amount of resistance can be increased or decreased by the trainer.
Coaching Points	This is a great strength-building exercise for those who are recovering from injury. Work with a qualified trainer or therapist who can determine the appropriate level of resistance.

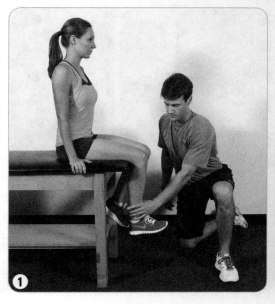

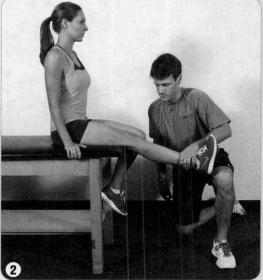

SINGLE-LEG EXTENSION

Target	Quads
When	End of the workout
Start	Adjust the back of the seat so that the axis of the machine is in line with your knee. Adjust the shin pad so that it is just above your ankle. Sit up straight with your back against the pad. Point your toes up.
Execution	Extend one leg slowly until it is just short of being locked. Return to the starting position in a slow and controlled manner.
Variations	This exercise can be done using negative training (placing heavy resistance on the eccentric portion of the lift). Extend the machine with both legs and resist the weight on the down, or lowering, phase with one leg. The opposite leg will rest during this time.
Coaching Points	Make sure you do not round your spine. Sit up tall. If you have a history of knee pain, limit your range of motion in the flexion phase of this exercise.

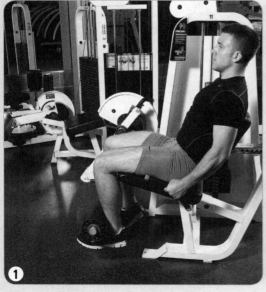

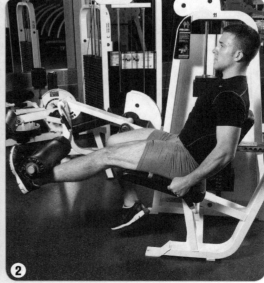

WALL SIT

Target	Quads
When	End of the workout
Start	Lean against a stable wall with your back, shoulders, and head against it. Keep your arms down at your sides.
Execution	Slide down the wall while maintaining contact with your head, back, and shoulders until your knees are flexed to 90 degrees. Hold this position in an isometric contraction for 1 to 2 minutes.
Variations	Hold a weighted plate or dumbbells for added resistance. For a very advanced move, try extending one leg while holding the original position with the other leg; this position increases the load on the muscles of the supporting leg.
Coaching Points	This is a great exercise for those who want to gain strength but have knee discomfort.

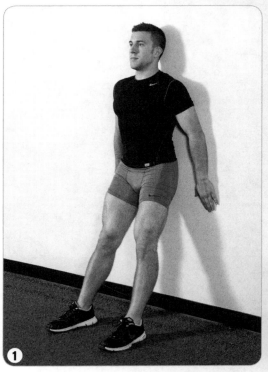

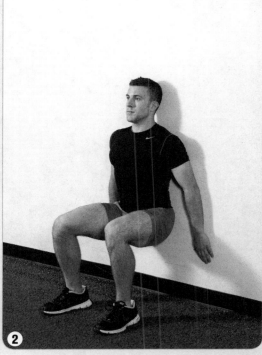

CHAPTER 6

Hamstring and Posterior Chain Exercises

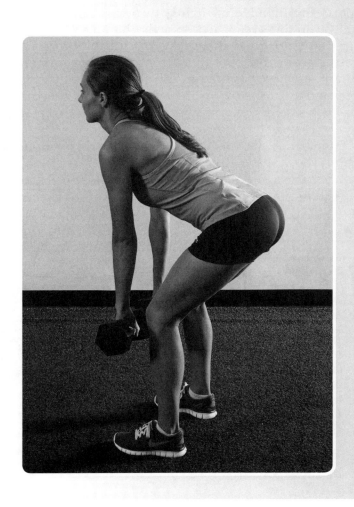

The hamstring muscles—the semitendinosus, the semimembranosus, and the biceps femoris—are located on the posterior thigh. They are responsible for bending and flexing the knee, and they also assist with hip extension. The hamstring group is often overlooked and undertrained. When people think about developing bigger and stronger legs, they usually think about the quads first. The hamstrings are hard to see, which leads to an "out of sight, out of mind" effect. But the quads are naturally stronger than the hamstrings because of their size and weight-bearing responsibility, so it is important to train the hamstrings as much or even more than the quads. A lack of strength in the hamstrings compared with the strength in the quads not only can create a cosmetic and functional imbalance, but it can also result in an unstable knee joint and assorted lower-body injuries.

The term *posterior chain* refers to the series of muscles that include the low back, the glutes, the hamstrings, and even the calf muscles. Posterior chain exercises involve most, if not all, of these muscles in a chainlike manner. Athletes in sports that involve swinging, throwing, and lifting know that generating power in one area is not enough; the muscles must be strong enough to transfer it along the chain.

Posterior chain exercises also contribute to a strong core. A common assumption is that the term *core* applies only to the abdominal muscles, but the low back, glutes, and even the top of the hamstrings are all part of the core as well. This back side of the core must also be developed and maintained.

Strong and flexible hamstrings and posterior chain muscles are an important part of an injury-prevention strategy. The low back is one of the most commonly injured areas, often leading to lost work hours and high medical expenses. And in the world of sports, athletes are routinely sidelined by hamstring injuries. Performing hamstring and posterior chain exercises can help you avoid becoming one of these statistics.

As with the quads and glutes, you can train the hamstring group and the posterior chain muscles by using compound movements such as deadlifts or isolation movements such as leg curls. You will see the best strength gains in this region of the body from using a combination of compound and isolation exercises.

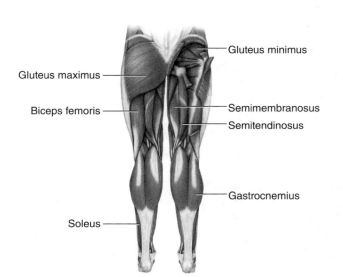

Gluteus minimus

Gluteus maximus

Biceps femoris

Semimembranosus

Semitendinosus

Gastrocnemius

Soleus

TRAP-BAR SQUAT

Target	Hamstrings, glutes, quads, calves, low back
When	Early in the workout
Start	Stand inside the trap bar with your feet shoulder-width apart. Squat down and grasp the center of the handles of the bar while maintaining a straight back. Keep your head up and looking forward.
Execution	Place the majority of your body weight toward your heels and then drive up while extending your ankles, knees, and hips. Keep your back straight (do not round at the shoulders) throughout the lift. Do not lock your knees at the top of the movement. Return slowly to the starting position.
Variations	You can place very small weight plates under your heels to shift the focus of the exercise more toward your quads.
Coaching Points	Maintain proper posture (back straight) throughout this exercise. Poor posture may lead to low back injury. Do not bounce the weight off the floor. If you can't control the weight and must bounce it to gain momentum, it is probably too heavy for you.

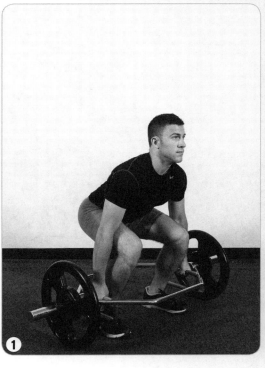

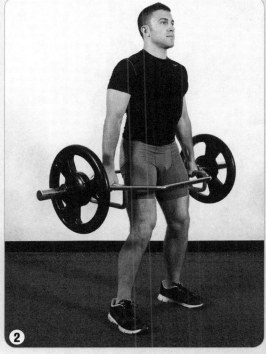

STRAIGHT-LEG DEADLIFT

Target	Hamstrings, glutes, low back
When	Early in the workout
Start	Stand with your feet hip-width apart. Hold a barbell with a shoulder-width overhand grip. Keep your knees locked and your shoulders back. Your head should be in a neutral position.
Execution	Flex at the hips by moving your buttocks backward. Lower the bar slowly toward your shins. Keep your shoulders drawn back with your back straight and head in the neutral position during the entire movement. Extend back up to the start position.
Variations	You can use dumbbells for this exercise. Using dumbbells does not significantly affect muscle involvement and may be more comfortable to use while learning the exercise. Hold one in each hand and follow the same execution as with a barbell.
Coaching Points	Focus on using your hamstrings to return to the upright position. Keep your back straight and shoulders back. Begin with a very light weight when learning this exercise. If you have any back pain or weakness, do not attempt this exercise.

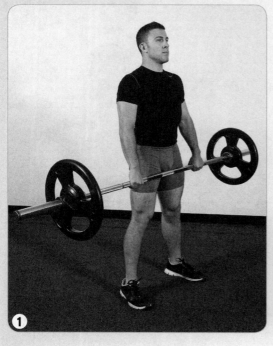

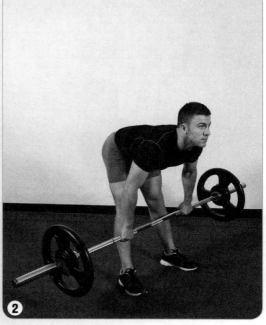

GOOD MORNING

Target	Hamstrings, glutes, low back
When	Early in the workout
Start	Stand with your feet about hip-width apart. Hold a barbell across your upper trap and lower shoulder muscles. Keep your knees locked and your shoulders back. Your head should be in a neutral position.
Execution	This is a difficult exercise. If you have back pain or weakness, do not attempt it. Flex at the hips by moving your buttocks backward. Lower the bar by slowly flexing forward at the hips. Keep your shoulders drawn back with your back straight and head in the neutral position during the entire movement. Stop when your upper body is about parallel to the floor. Extend back up to the start position.
Variations	You may find it more comfortable to keep a slight bend in the knees. This reduces the effect on the hamstrings somewhat, but it puts less pressure on your low back.
Coaching Points	Focus on using your hamstrings to return to the upright position. Keep your back straight and shoulders back. Never round or twist your back during the movement. Begin with a very light weight when learning this exercise.

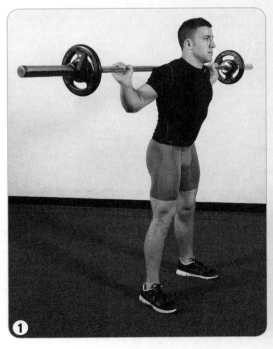
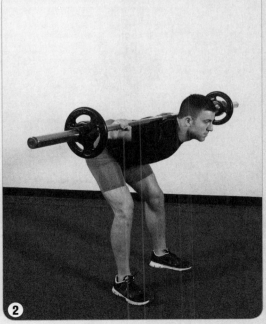

ROMANIAN DEADLIFT

Target	Hamstrings, glutes, calves
When	Early in the workout
Start	Stand with your feet about hip-width apart. Hold a barbell with a shoulder-width overhand grip. Keep a slight bend in your knees and your shoulders back. Your head should be in a neutral position.
Execution	Flex at the hips by moving your buttocks backward. Lower the bar slowly toward your shins. Keep your shoulders drawn back, your back straight, and your head in the neutral position during the entire movement. Extend back up to the start position.
Variations	You can use dumbbells for this exercise. Hold one in each hand and follow the same execution as with a barbell. Using dumbbells will not have a significantly different impact on the muscles involved, but they may be easier for some people to handle when learning the exercise.
Coaching Points	Focus on using your hamstrings to return to the upright position. Always keep a slight bend in your knees with your back straight and shoulders back. Begin with a very light weight when learning this exercise.

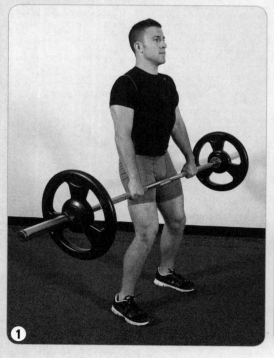

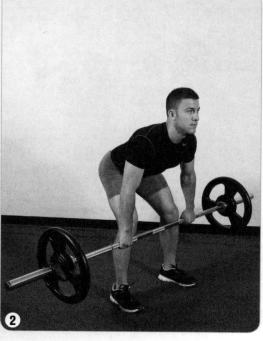

SINGLE-LEG SINGLE-ARM ROMANIAN DEADLIFT

Target	Hamstrings, glutes, calves, low back
When	Middle of the workout
Start	Stand with your feet about hip-width apart. Hold a dumbbell in one hand with an overhand grip. Keep a slight bend in your knees and your shoulders back. Your head should be in a neutral position.
Execution	Flex at the hips by moving your buttocks backward. Lift the leg on the dumbbell side of the body. Lower the dumbbell slowly to about shin level, keeping your shoulders drawn back with your back straight and head in the neutral position for the entire movement. Extend back up to the start position.
Variations	You can use a smaller straight bar for this exercise as well. Using a bar slightly increases the involvement of the muscles used to maintain balance.
Coaching Points	Focus on using your hamstrings to return to the upright position. Always keep a slight bend in your knee with your back straight and shoulders back. Keep your torso level and avoid leaning too much to the side where the weight is. Begin with a very light weight when learning this exercise.

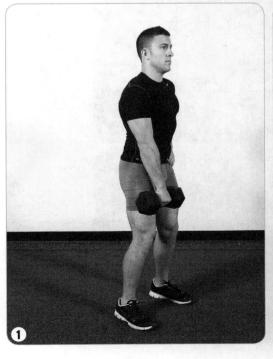

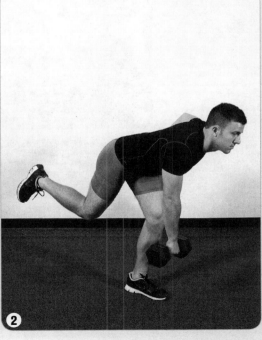

PRONE LEG CURL

Target   Hamstrings, glutes

When   Middle of the workout

Start   Lie in the prone position on a leg-curl machine with your knees just beyond the end of the bench. Place the pad of the machine just above your ankles. Make sure the cam of the machine is in line with your knees.

Execution   Flex your legs at the knees and raise the pad of the machine toward your glutes. Hold for one count and slowly lower to the start position.

Variations   There are numerous leg-curl machines (including seated leg-curl machines) that you can use to add variation. Each type of machine works the muscles in a slightly different way; use whichever position is comfortable for you.

Coaching Points Make sure you keep your spine in a neutral position. Do not lift off the machine with your hips. If you cannot hold your hips down, you are probably using too much weight.

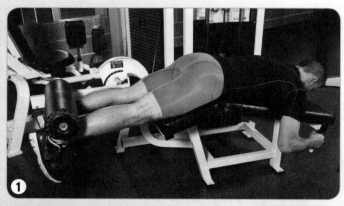

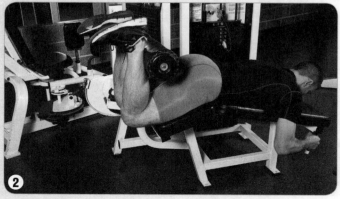

SINGLE-LEG TOE TOUCH

Target Hamstrings, glutes, hip flexors, calves

When Middle of the workout

Start Stand on one leg with a slight bend in the knee. Draw your shoulders back and keep your head in a neutral position. Keep your non-weight-bearing leg in front of you with your hip and knee flexed. Keep your hands out in front of your body.

Execution Bend forward at the hips with your back straight and head up. Extend your non-weight-bearing leg behind you while maintaining the flex in the knee. Reach down toward your toes, stopping about shin level. Return to the starting position by extending at the hips and bringing your non-weight-bearing leg forward again with the knee and hip flexed.

Variations To add resistance, hold a medicine ball with both hands or stand on a half foam roller.

Coaching Points Keep the back straight at all times, while maintaining a slight natural curvature in your low back. If you lose your balance, simply tap your non-weight-bearing foot to the floor until you are back under control. Do not hop or swing your arms in an attempt to regain your balance.

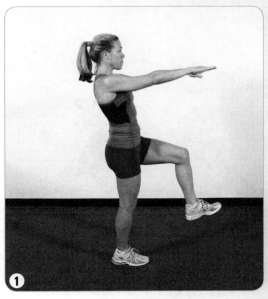

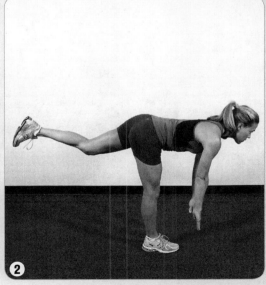

HAMSTRING LOWER

Target	Hamstrings, glutes, calves
When	Middle of the workout
Start	While kneeling, place your heels underneath a secure object (or have a partner hold on to your lower legs just above the ankles), with your knees bent at 90 degrees.
Execution	Slowly lower your upper body toward the floor with your hands out in front of you. Resist your body weight by eccentrically contracting your hamstrings. Once your hands hit the floor, push yourself back up to the starting position.
Variations	Place a box or a bench in front of you to limit the range of motion if necessary.
Coaching Points	This is a very difficult exercise. Begin with a limited range of motion and then work your way up to going all the way to the floor. For added safety and comfort, do this exercise on a mat.

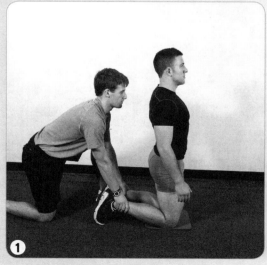
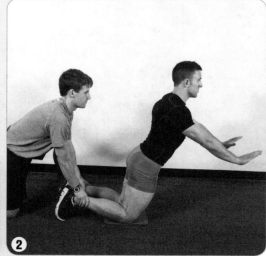

DOUBLE-LEG STRAIGHT-LEG BRIDGE

Target   Hamstrings, glutes, calves, low back

When   Late in the workout

Start   Lie on your back with your legs straight and your arms at your sides. Place your heels on an exercise bench or 12-inch box (30 cm).

Execution   Raise your hips off the floor by contracting your glutes and hamstrings and driving your heels into the bench or box. Stop the movement once your spine is in a neutral position. Return slowly to the start position.

Variations   You can perform this movement with your heels on an exercise ball. This will increase the amount of stabilization needed in the core area.

Coaching Points   Do not push into the floor with your head, neck, or arms. Stop the movement as soon as your spine is in a neutral position. Do not hyperextend your back. Make sure your heels are securely on the bench, box, or ball.

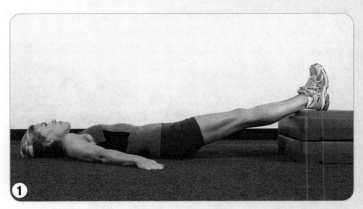

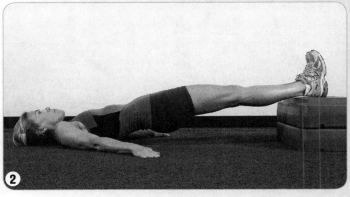

SINGLE-LEG STRAIGHT-LEG BRIDGE

Target	Hamstrings, glutes, calves, low back
When	Late in the workout
Start	Lie on your back with your legs straight and your arms at your sides. Place one heel on an exercise bench or 12-inch box (30 cm). Keep the opposite leg straight and slightly higher than the involved leg.
Execution	Raise your hips off the floor by contracting your glutes and hamstrings and driving your heel into the bench or box. Stop the movement once your spine is in a neutral position. Return slowly to the start position.
Variations	You can perform this movement with your heel on an exercise ball. This will add a great deal of intensity to the hamstring and will increase the amount of stabilization needed in the core area.
Coaching Points	Do not push into the floor with your head, neck, or arms. Stop the movement as soon as your spine is in a neutral position. Do not hyperextend your back. Make sure your heel is securely on the bench, box, or ball.

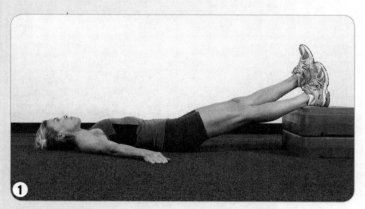

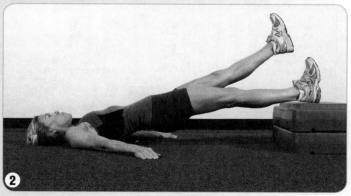

DOUBLE-LEG FLEXED-LEG BRIDGE

Target
Hamstrings, glutes, calves, low back

When
Late in the workout

Start
Lie on your back with your legs bent to 90 degrees and arms at your sides. Place your heels on an exercise bench or 12-inch box (30 cm).

Execution
Raise your hips off the floor by contracting your glutes and hamstrings and driving your heels into the bench or box. Maintain the 90-degree flex in your legs during the exercise. Stop the movement once your spine is in a neutral position. Return slowly to the start position.

Variations
You can perform this exercise with your heels on an exercise ball. This will increase the amount of stabilization needed in the core area.

Coaching Points
Do not push into the floor with your head, neck, or arms. Stop the movement as soon as your spine is in a neutral position. Do not hyperextend your back. Make sure your heels are securely on the bench, box, or ball.

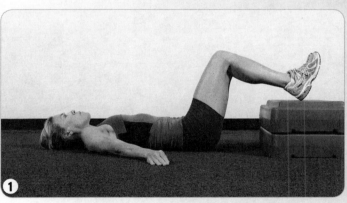

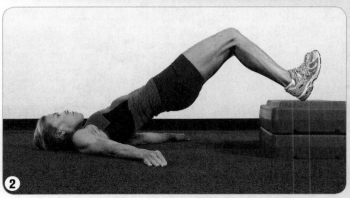

SINGLE-LEG FLEXED-LEG BRIDGE

Target	Hamstrings, glutes, calves, low back
When	Late in the workout
Start	Lie on your back with your legs bent to 90 degrees and arms at your sides. Place one heel on an exercise bench or 12-inch box (30 cm). Straighten the opposite leg and raise it slightly higher than the involved leg.
Execution	Raise your hips off the floor by contracting your glutes and hamstrings and driving your heel into the bench or box. Maintain the 90-degree flex in your leg during the exercise. Stop the movement once your spine is in a neutral position. Return slowly to the start position.
Variations	You can perform this exercise with your heel on an exercise ball. This will add intensity to the hamstrings and challenge the core to stabilize more throughout the exercise.
Coaching Points	Do not push into the floor with your head, neck, or arms. Stop the movement as soon as your spine is in a neutral position. Do not hyperextend your back. Make sure your heel is securely on the bench, box, or ball.

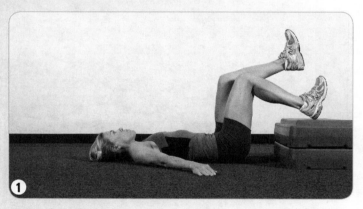

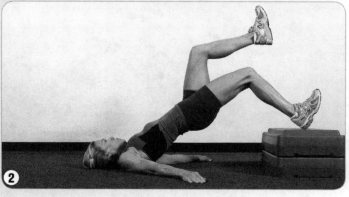

ROMAN CHAIR HIP EXTENSION

Target	Hamstrings, glutes, low back
When	Late in the workout
Start	Lie prone on the chair with the pads at hip level. Secure your feet under the foot pads while keeping your feet flat on the platform. Place your arms across your chest.
Execution	Extend upward slowly by contracting the muscles in the low back, glutes, and hamstrings. Raise your upper body until your spine is in a neutral position. Do not hyperextend your back. Pause for one second at the top and return slowly to the starting position.
Variations	Holding a weight plate or medicine ball will add intensity to the exercise by increasing the amount of stabilization needed in the core area.
Coaching Points	Keep your back flat with your head and neck in a neutral position. Be very careful not to hyperextend your back at the top of the movement.

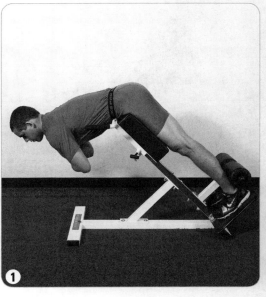

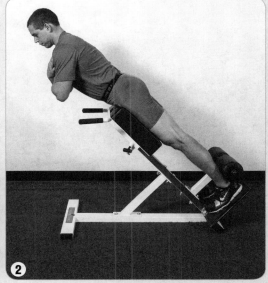

ROMAN CHAIR SINGLE-LEG HIP EXTENSION

Target   Hamstrings, glutes, low back

When   Late in the workout

Start   Lie prone on the chair with the pads at hip level. Secure one foot under the foot pad and flat on the platform, while keeping the opposite foot free from the platform. Place your arms across your chest.

Execution   Extend upward slowly by contracting the muscles in the low back, glutes, and hamstrings. Raise your upper body until your spine is in a neutral position. Do not hyperextend your back. Pause for one second at the top and return slowly to the starting position.

Variations   Holding a weight plate or medicine ball will add intensity to the exercise by increasing the amount of stabilization needed in the core area..

Coaching Points Keep your back flat with your head and neck in a neutral position. This is a difficult movement that requires strength and balance. Begin with fewer reps and increase as you get stronger.

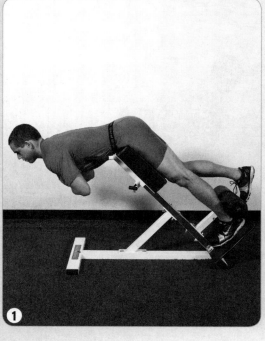

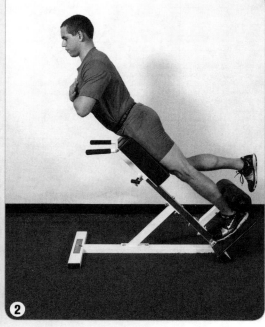

PRONE NEGATIVE LEG CURL

Target Hamstrings, glutes

When Late in the workout

Start Lie in the prone position on a leg-curl machine with your knees just off the end of the bench. Place the pad of the machine just above your ankles. Make sure the cam of the machine is in line with your knees.

Execution Your partner assists you in lifting the arm of the leg-curl machine until you have flexed your knees at least 90 degrees. Your partner lets go of the arm of the machine at this point. Hold for one count and lower slowly to the start position.

Variations You can perform this exercise using a single leg as well. A single-leg curl adds intensity and encourages a balance of strength in both legs.

Coaching Points You may be able to use slightly higher weights than you normally use on your standard leg-curl movement. Begin increasing the weight gradually. Do not go directly to significantly heavier weights.

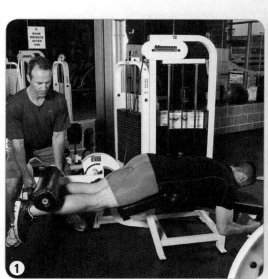

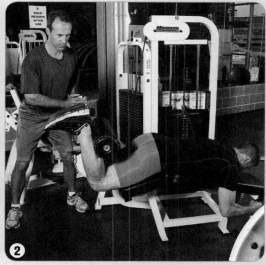

MANUAL-RESISTANCE PRONE LEG CURL

Target   Hamstrings, glutes

When   Late in the workout

Start   Lie in the prone position on a training table with your legs straight and knees just off the end of the table. Keep your toes pointing straight down toward the floor.

Execution   Your trainer or training partner grasps one leg just below the calf and just above the heel. Flex the involved leg against the resistance of your partner. Proceed until your heel is close to your buttocks. Return to the starting position by resisting your partner in the eccentric, or negative, direction.

Variations   The resistance can be increased or decreased by your partner. The speed of the movement may also be manipulated by your partner; increasing the velocity of the movement creates a more ballistic movement. This may be appropriate for those recovering from an injury and who are trying to get back into running or another activity that involves quick movements.

Coaching Points Communication is the key to this exercise. You must talk to your partner throughout this exercise to get and maintain the proper resistance. If you are unable to finish the recommended reps during a given set while keeping proper form, the resistance given by your partner may be too great. Always begin with lighter resistance and then work your way up to heavier resistance. If you are able to complete the prescribed number of reps without a challenge, your partner should increase the resistance.

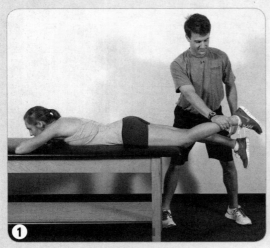
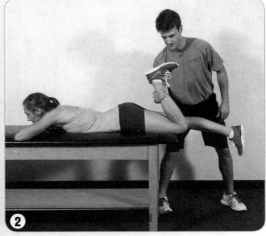

FUNCTIONAL-TRAINER LEG CURL

Target	Hamstrings, glutes
When	Late in the workout
Start	Attach the strap to your lower leg just above the ankle. Hook the functional-trainer cable to the front of the strap while facing the machine. Stand on a 6-inch box (15 cm) with the nonworking leg and balance yourself by holding onto the machine.
Execution	Flex your working leg at the knee, bringing your heel toward your buttocks. Return to the starting position by slowly resisting the weight of the machine.
Variations	You may add a half foam roller under your uninvolved foot to increase the difficulty of the exercise.
Coaching Points	Be careful not to sway at the hips. Maintain proper posture throughout the exercise.

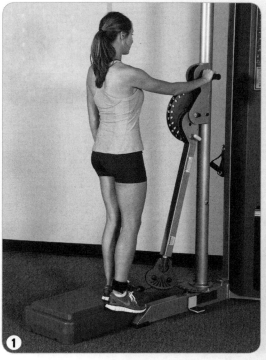
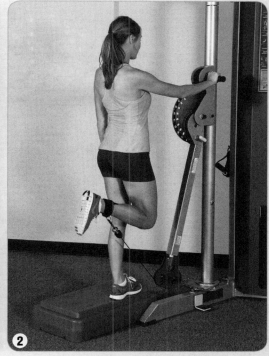

EXERCISE-BALL SUPINE LEG CURL

Target	Hamstrings, glutes, calves
When	Late in the workout
Start	Lie on your back with your arms at your sides and your heels resting on top of an exercise ball. Keep your legs straight and toes pointing up.
Execution	Press your heels into the ball while raising your hips off the floor. Flex your knees and bring your heels in toward your buttocks while keeping your hips elevated. Return to the starting position by extending your knees.
Variations	You can do this exercise with a single leg. Hold the uninvolved leg at 90 degrees and in an elevated position off the ball while performing the exercise with the opposite leg. This variation works the hamstrings harder and engages the core stabilizers.
Coaching Points	Be careful not to press down into the floor with your head and neck. Make sure the hips remain elevated throughout the entire movement. Attempt the single-leg curl *only* after you've mastered the double-leg curl.

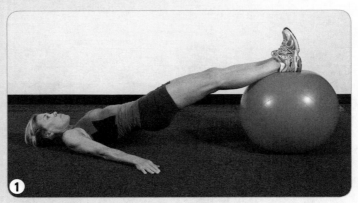

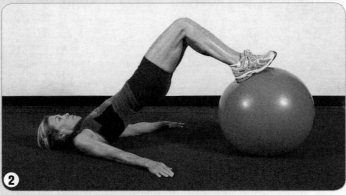

SLIDE SUPINE LEG CURL

Target   Hamstrings, glutes, calves

When   Late in the workout

Start   Lie on your back with your arms at your sides. Place the heels of your feet directly in the middle of the slide with your toes pointing up. Slide your feet in toward your buttocks by flexing your knees.

Execution Press down through your heels and contract your glutes to lift your hips off the floor until your spine is in a neutral position. Slowly slide your feet away from your buttocks by extending your legs. Go until your legs are almost straight. Return to the starting position by contracting your hamstrings and glutes while flexing your knees. Keep your hips off the floor during the entire movement. If cramping occurs during the flexion portion of the exercise, perform the extension phase only (see variation).

Variations Because of the intensity of this exercise, beginners should start with the negative (extending the knees) phase of this exercise only. After each extension, drop your hips to the floor and slide your feet back toward your buttocks. Lift your hips back up and repeat.

Coaching Points This is a very aggressive and difficult exercise. Stop the exercise immediately if you sense that your muscles are starting to cramp during the flexion portion of the movement and return to performing only the extension phase described in the variation section.

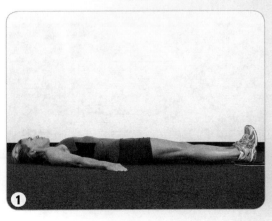
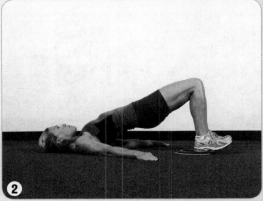

PRONE SINGLE-LEG CURL

Target   Hamstrings, glutes

When   End of the workout

Start   Lie in the prone position on a leg-curl machine with your knees just off the end of the bench. Place the pad of the machine just above your ankles. Make sure the cam of the machine is in line with your knee.

Execution   Flex one leg at the knee and raise the pad of the machine toward your glutes. Hold for one count and slowly lower to the start position.

Variations   There are some machines that will allow you to perform this exercise while standing. This change in position will slightly change the way the muscle is worked and may be more comfortable for some individuals.

Coaching Points   Make sure you keep your spine in a neutral position. Do not lift off the machine with your hips. If you cannot hold your hips down, you are probably using too much weight. You may also have a tendency to lean to one side when performing the single-leg curl because of the overload and imbalance of weight being placed on just one leg. Avoid twisting your spine.

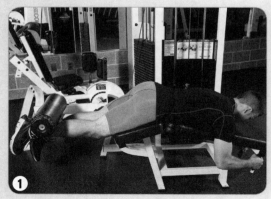

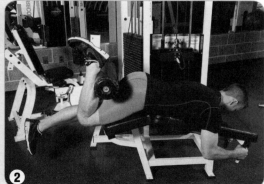

CHAPTER 7

Lower-Leg
Exercises

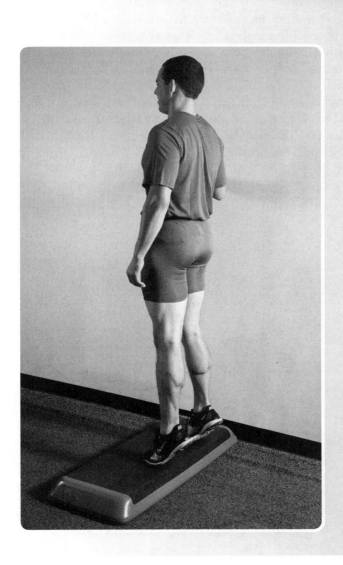

The two main muscles of the posterior lower leg, or the calf, are the gastrocnemius and the soleus. The soleus lies beneath the more visible gastrocnemius and is much smaller. These muscles are responsible for plantar flexion (pressing the toes downward and elevating the heel). Plantar flexion is critical in many athletic movements, especially sprinting, jumping, and even recreational jogging. The soleus is called upon for plantar flexion when the knee is bent as in seated calf raises; the gastrocnemius is recruited when the leg is extended as in standing calf raises. Both of these muscles attach to the heel via the Achilles tendon, which tends to become weaker and less flexible as we age. Strengthening the muscles that surround the Achilles tendon can help prevent injury and promote good range of motion during sport and other recreational activities.

The antagonist of the gastrocnemius and the soleus is the tibialis anterior. The tibialis anterior is responsible for the dorsiflexion and inversion of the ankle that occurs in exercises like the heel walk. The tibialis anterior also helps stabilize the ankle during foot contact with the ground. Because many machines and exercises are geared to the gastrocnemius and the soleus, the tibialis muscle is often overlooked in training programs. However, many of the exercises provided in this chapter are designed to strengthen it.

While the calf muscles and the tibialis anterior are used during compound exercises, they are trained more effectively using isolation movements. The ankle is the only joint that is involved during most of the lower leg exercises; therefore compound movements, such as those in the exercises in chapters 4, 5, and 6, are not typically used to gain strength in the lower legs.

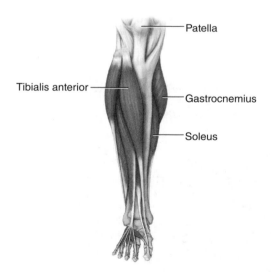

LEG-PRESS CALF RAISE

Target	Gastrocnemius
When	Late in the workout
Start	Place the balls of your feet on the edge of a leg-press platform. Keep your legs straight but not locked out. Keep your back flat and your hips down against the pad.
Execution	Press the balls of your feet (ankles plantar flexed) into the platform of the leg press by moving only at the ankles. Pause for one count at the top of the movement and then return slowly to the starting position.
Variations	You can work the calf muscle in a functionally different way by varying your foot placement on the platform, slightly turning your toes in or out. You may also perform this exercise with one leg to increase the intensity and force the muscles to work to maintain balance.
Coaching Points	Be very careful when using the leg-press machine for this exercise. If your feet are not securely on the edge of the platform, they may slip. Make sure you use the safety catches on the machine to avoid injury.

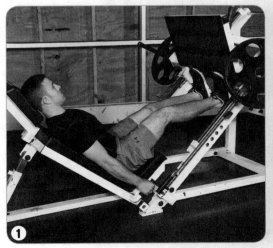

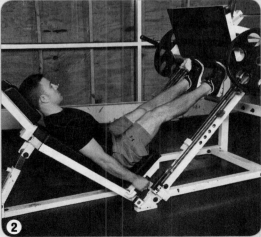

LEG-SLED CALF RAISE

Target	Gastrocnemius
When	Late in the workout
Start	Place the balls of your feet on the edge of a leg-sled platform. Keep your legs straight but not locked out. Keep your back flat and your hips down against the pad.
Execution	Press the balls of your feet (plantar flex) into the platform by moving only at the ankles. Pause for one count at the top of the movement and then return slowly to the starting position.
Variations	You can work the calf muscle in a functionally different way by varying your foot placement on the platform, slightly turning your toes in or out. You may also perform this exercise with one leg to add intensity and force the muscles to work to maintain balance.
Coaching Points	Be very careful when using the leg-press sled machine for this exercise. Make sure your feet are securely on the platform. Injury may occur if your feet slip off the machine during the exercise.

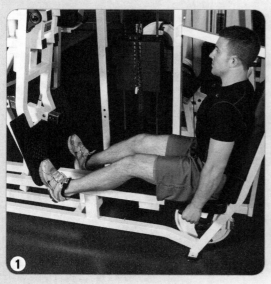 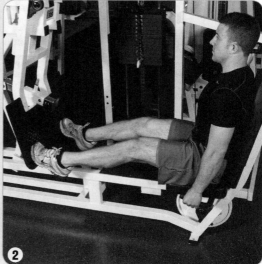

STANDING CALF RAISE

Target	Gastrocnemius
When	Late in the workout
Start	Stand with the balls of your feet on the edge of a 6-inch step (15 cm). Lightly balance yourself with your hands on a wall or stable object. Begin with your ankles dorsiflexed and legs straight but not completely locked out.
Execution	Push up onto the balls of your feet by plantar flexing your ankles. Hold for one count at the top and then slowly return to the starting position by resisting your body weight.
Variations	You can perform this exercise without a step while holding a straight bar for added resistance. You may also perform this exercise with one foot on the step to add intensity and make the muscles work to maintain balance. Wear a weighted vest or hold a dumbbell in the opposite hand for added resistance on the single-leg calf raise.
Coaching Points	You may have a tendency to go too fast during this exercise. Make sure you move in a slow, controlled manner.

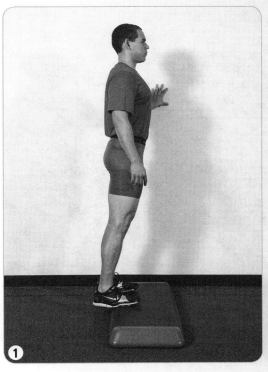 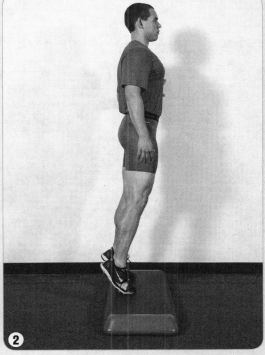

MACHINE STANDING CALF RAISE

Target	Gastrocnemius
When	Late in the workout
Start	Stand on the platform with the balls of your feet. Lightly hold the grips of the machine. Begin with your ankles dorsiflexed and legs straight but not completely locked.
Execution	Push up onto the balls of your feet by plantar flexing your ankles. Hold for one count at the top and then slowly return to the starting position by resisting the weight of the machine.
Variations	You may change your foot placement on the platform to work the involved muscles in a slightly different manner.
Coaching Points	You may have a tendency to go too fast during this exercise. Make sure you move in a slow, controlled manner. Also be careful not to hyperextend your back during this movement. Keep your spine in a neutral position throughout the exercise.

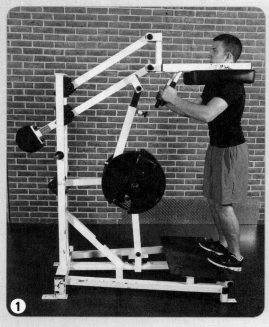 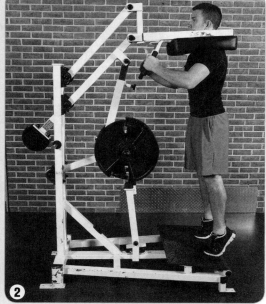

FUNCTIONAL-TRAINER STANDING CALF RAISE

Target
Gastrocnemius

When
Late in the workout

Start
Stand with the ball of one foot on the edge of a 6-inch step (15 cm). Balance yourself by holding onto the functional trainer. Hold the handle of the functional trainer in the opposite hand. Begin with your ankle dorsiflexed and legs straight but not completely locked.

Execution
Push up onto the ball of your foot by plantar flexing your ankle. Hold for one count at the top and then slowly return to the starting position by resisting the weight.

Variations
You may perform this exercise with both legs, allowing you to use heavier weight. Hold both handles and remove the step before execution. Do not attempt this exercise using both hands and both legs while using the step.

Coaching Points
Maintain an upright posture throughout this exercise. You may have a tendency to go too fast during this exercise. Make sure you move in a slow, controlled manner.

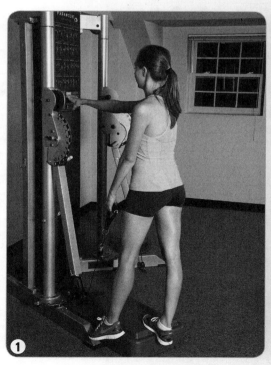
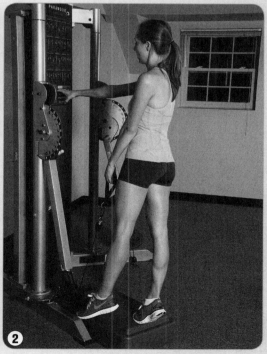

MACHINE SEATED CALF RAISE

Target	Soleus
When	Late in the workout
Start	Sit on the calf-raise machine with upright posture and the balls of your feet on the foot support. Begin with your ankles dorsiflexed. The padded arm of the machine should rest on your lower quads.
Execution	Push up onto the balls of your feet by plantar flexing your ankles. Hold for one count at the top and then slowly return to the starting position by resisting the weight.
Variations	You can work the calf muscle in a functionally different way by varying your foot placement on the platform, slightly turning your toes in or out.
Coaching Points	Make sure the balls of your feet remain on the platform at all times. They may have a tendency to slip during the exercise. Do not rock your upper body in order to gain momentum while raising the weight.

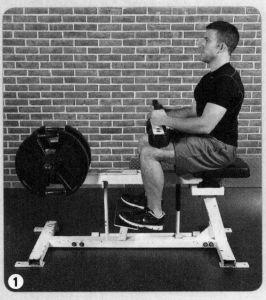
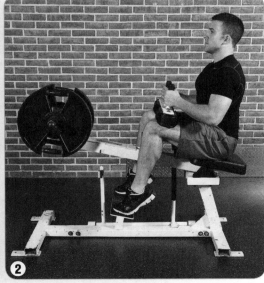

SEATED CALF RAISE

Target	Soleus
When	Late in the workout
Start	Sit on the end of a bench with upright posture and place the balls of your feet on a 2-inch by 4-inch board (5 by 10 cm), a 6-inch step (15 cm), or weight plates. Begin with your ankles dorsiflexed. Hold a dumbbell in the upright position on each lower thigh.
Execution	Push up onto the balls of your feet by plantar flexing your ankles. Hold for one count at the top and then slowly return to the starting position by resisting the weight.
Variations	You can vary your foot placement on the board, step, or weight plate by slightly turning your toes in or out. This will work the calf muscle in a functionally different way. You may also hold a straight bar with weight plates across both lower thighs for added resistance.
Coaching Points	Make sure the balls of your feet remain on the board, step, or weight plates at all times. They may have a tendency to slip throughout the exercise. Do not rock your upper body in order to gain momentum while raising the weight.

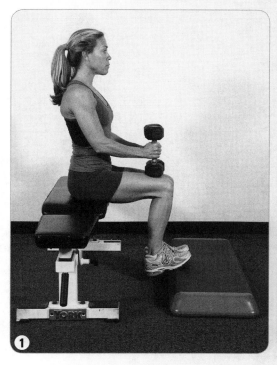
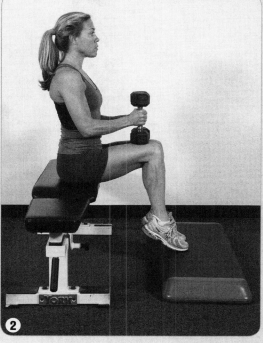

DYNAMIC AXIAL RESISTANCE DEVICE (DARD) RAISE

Target	Tibialis anterior
When	Late in the workout
Start	Sit upright on the end of a bench or training table. You should be elevated high enough so that your feet do not touch the floor. Place the pads of the DARD on the upper portion of your feet.
Execution	Dorsiflex your feet against the resistance of the device. Pause for one count at the top and return slowly to the starting position.
Variations	You can try this exercise using only one foot for added challenge. Balancing is difficult, however, so you will have to use very light weight.
Coaching Points	Do not overdo this exercise, especially when you are first trying it. Start with light weight and only a few reps and work your way up.

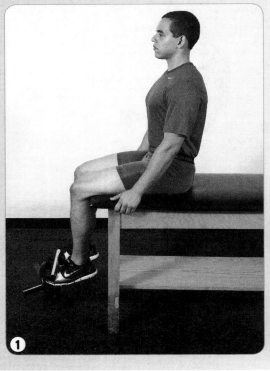
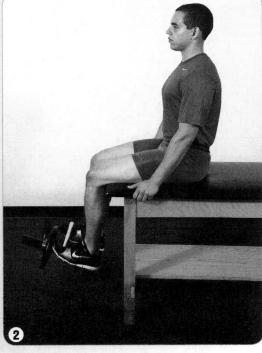

RESISTANCE-BAND DORSIFLEXION

Target	Tibialis anterior
When	Late in the workout
Start	Secure a piece of resistance band or tubing around a sturdy table or bench. Place the tubing or band around the upper foot of one leg. Keep the opposite leg bent with your foot flat on the floor. Move away from the table or bench to create tension on the band.
Execution	Begin with your ankle in a plantar-flexed position. Slowly dorsiflex your ankle, working against the resistance of the band. Hold for one count at the top position and then return to the starting position.
Variations	You can use various strengths of resistance bands to increase or decrease the amount of resistance.
Coaching Points	Make sure the band is secure. It may have a tendency to move so recheck the position after a few repetitions.

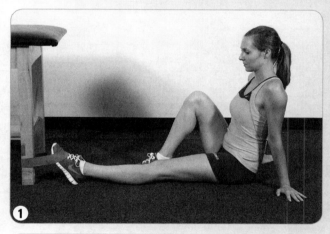

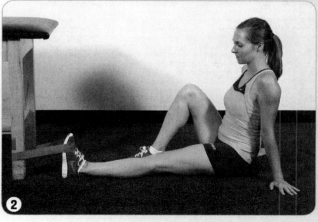

FUNCTIONAL-TRAINER DORSIFLEXION

Target   Tibialis anterior

When   Late in the workout

Start   Secure a strap around your foot and attach it to the machine. Keep the opposite leg bent with your foot flat on the floor. Move away from the machine to create tension on the cable.

Execution   Begin with your ankle in a plantar-flexed position. Slowly dorsiflex your ankle, working against the resistance of the weight stack. Hold for one count at the top position and then return to the starting position.

Variations   You can perform this exercise using any type of pulley system; use whatever available system appeals to you. The calibration may vary from system to system.

Coaching Points   Make sure you move only at the ankle joint. If your knee is bending, you are probably using too much weight.

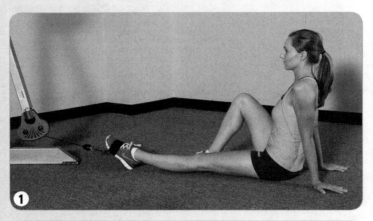

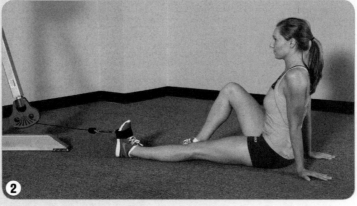

WEIGHT-PLATE SEATED DORSIFLEXION

Target Tibialis anterior

When Late in the workout

Start Sit upright on the end of a bench with your knees bent at 90 degrees and your feet flat on the floor. Rest an individual weight plate (the flat side) on the top of each foot (about half of the plate will be on your foot and half off your foot).

Execution Raise your toes up by dorsiflexing your ankles. Hold for one count at the top and then return slowly to the starting position.

Variations Various types of plates work for this exercise; you can use whatever is available at your facility. Plates with at least one flat side are best.

Coaching Points Make sure you are moving only at the ankle. You should not have any movement at the knee. Begin lightly (using 5 to 10 lb) and progress to heavier weight (up to 25 lb).

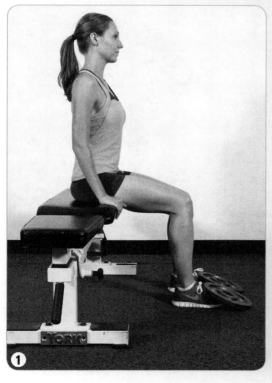
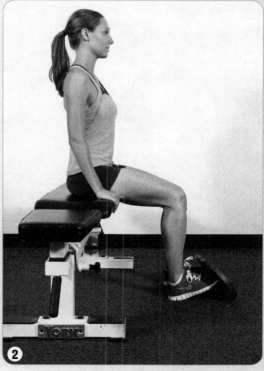

HEEL WALK

Target	Tibialis anterior
When	Late in the workout
Start	Stand tall with your toes pointing up and your ankles dorsiflexed.
Execution	Walk on your heels while in the dorsiflexed position. Take normal-length strides.
Variations	You can do this exercise on a treadmill as well as on the floor. A treadmill may have a surer surface and allow you to do more repetitions within your allotted area.
Coaching Points	Keep a slight bend in your knees during the exercise. Start with a short distance (5 to 10 yds or 4 to 9 m) and work your way up to longer distances (20 to 30 yds or 18 to 27 m).

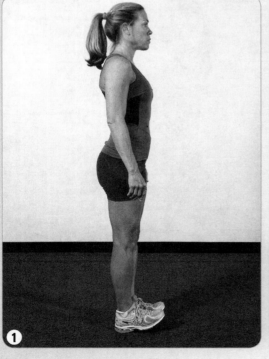

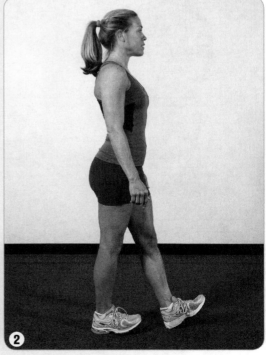

FUNCTIONAL-TRAINER HIP FLEXION WITH DORSIFLEXION

Target	Tibialis anterior, hip flexors
When	Late in the workout
Start	Sit up tall on the end of a bench or chair with an appropriate strap placed around your foot (preferably a strap with a hook that attaches underneath the foot to the functional trainer). Hook the cable to the strap with your foot in a dorsiflexed position. Keep the opposite knee at 90 degrees with the foot flat on the floor.
Execution	Flex your hip and bring your knee toward your chest while maintaining flexion in your ankle. Hold for one count at the top of the movement and then slowly lower your foot to the starting position.
Variations	You can do this exercise with resistance bands instead of the machine to increase resistance.
Coaching Points	Do not lean back or rock during the movement. If you cannot maintain your posture, the weight is probably too heavy.

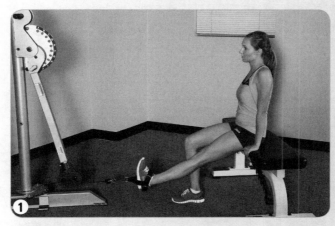

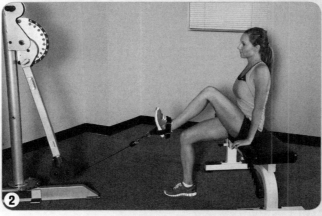

STANDING DORSIFLEXION

Target	Tibialis anterior
When	Late in the workout
Start	Stand with your heels on the edge of a 6-inch box (15 cm) or step, your toes pointing down toward the floor. Balance yourself against a stable object.
Execution	Dorsiflex your feet until your toes are as high as you can raise them. Hold for one count and then return to the starting position.
Variations	This exercise can be performed by standing on a weight plate or other stable object if there is no box available.
Coaching Points	Be very careful you do not slip off the box or step. You may have to adjust your feet every couple of reps to prevent your heels from slipping off the step.

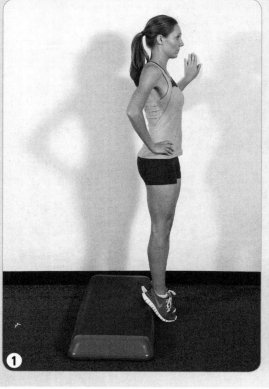
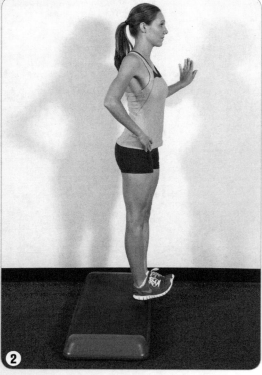

RESISTANCE-BAND INVERSION

Target   Tibialis anterior, tibialis posterior

When   Late in workout

Start   While seated on the floor, place the resistance band around your foot and secure the other end to a heavy table or bench.

Execution   Invert the foot (turn the foot so that the sole of the foot faces inward) against the resistance of the band. Hold the position for one count and then return slowly to the start.

Variations   You can use a cable for this exercise; the degree of resistance may vary slightly.

Coaching Points Focus the movement only at the ankle. If your leg moves at the hip, the resistance is probably too great.

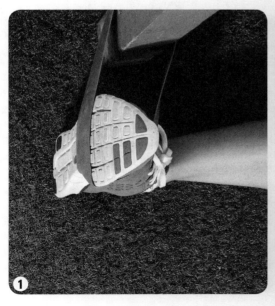

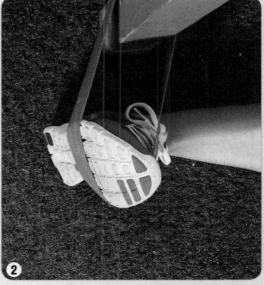

RESISTANCE-BAND SEATED DORSIFLEXION

Target	Tibialis anterior, hip flexors
When	Late in the workout
Start	While seated on a bench or box, place a loop of resistance band or tubing around your working foot and secure the other end by placing it under the other foot.
Execution	Flex your hip and pull the knee of the working leg toward your chest. From this position, dorsiflex your foot (bring toes toward your shin) and return slowly to the start. Repeat on the opposite foot.
Variations	You can use various levels of resistance bands or tubing for this exercise to change the intensity.
Coaching Points	Focus movement only at the ankle and hip. If your upper body moves, the resistance is probably too great. Make sure the resistance band is securely around your foot.

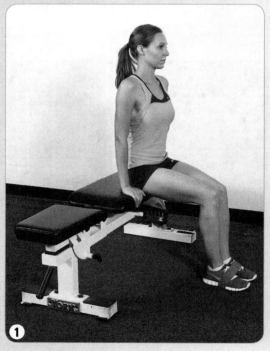
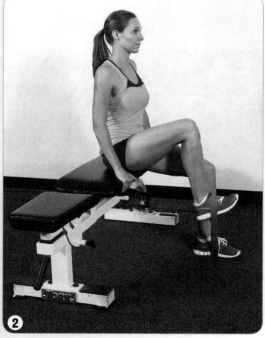

CHAPTER 8

Explosive Multijoint Exercises

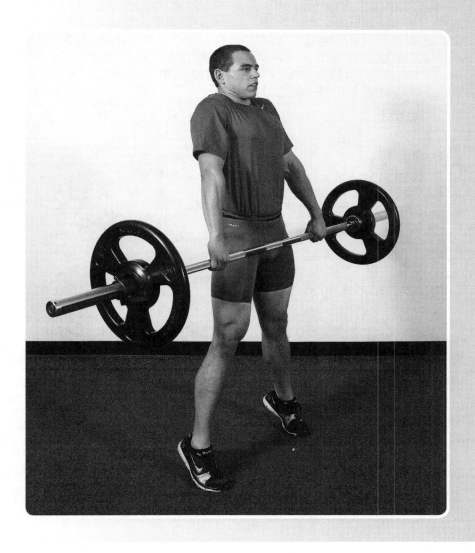

Explosive multijoint exercises are ideal if you want to increase strength and power. Because power may be defined as the rate at which work (in this case the lift) is done, the speed at which the multijoint explosive exercises are done is very important. For example, the hang clean must be performed in an explosive fashion. During the pull phase, the rapid extension of the ankles, knees, and hips creates an upward force on the barbell. This momentum allows the bar to continue to travel upward as the lifter releases the barbell and prepares for the catch phase. Performing this exercise at a slow pace would not be effective.

The rapid extension of the ankles, knees, and hips makes it difficult to pinpoint a single muscle group that is more dominant than another. The quads (rectus femoris, vastus intermedius, vastus medialis, and vastus lateralis); the hamstrings (semitendinosus, semimembranosus, and biceps femoris); the glutes (gluteus maximus, gluteus medius, gluteus minimus); the calves (gastrocnemius and soleus); and the adductor group (adductor brevis, adductor longus, and adductor magnus) are responsible for these compound exercises. (See chapter 1 for more information on the location and function of these muscles.)

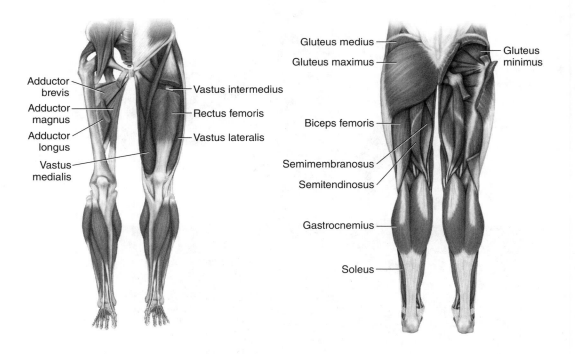

The muscles of the low back, the upper back, and even the shoulders are supporting muscle groups that assist with extending the spine and shrugging the shoulders. For instance, during the final pull of the power clean exercise, the shrug of the shoulders is a necessary link in the power chain to keep the momentum of the bar moving upward. The traps and other upper body muscles, along with the middle and low back, act as stabilizers during explosive multijoint exercises. Because they work so many muscle groups, explosive multijoint exercises increase total body strength and power. They also add variety to a program and can help increase strength in specific muscle groups.

It is no wonder that these exercises are very popular with athletes, including those who want to gain strength without adding body mass, such as wrestlers, gymnasts, and runners. The strength gains stem primarily from the increased motor unit recruitment and firing rate involved in these lifts and not from increased cross-sectional muscle area.

Multijoint exercises are very functional in nature. They help develop tremendous power because of their explosiveness. They also develop strength because of the heavy loads that are being lifted.

POWER CLEAN

Target
Glutes, quads, hamstrings, gastrocnemius and soleus, traps and delts

When
Early in the workout

Start
Stand with the balls of your feet under the bar, feet slightly more than hip-width apart. Squat down and grip the bar with an overhand grip slightly more than shoulder-width apart. Your arms should be outside your knees and straight, with your elbows pointing out. Keep your head up (in a neutral position with the spine) with your chest out and shoulders pulled back. Position your shoulders over the bar with your back straight or slightly arched.

Execution
Initial Pull: Begin the power clean by lifting the bar off the floor by extending your knees and hips. (Make sure your hips and shoulders move at the same time and at the same pace). Keep your head in the neutral position with your back straight and arms fully extended as you pull the bar up as close to your shins as you can.

Transition Phase: Drive your hips forward and move your body weight more toward the front of your feet. Do not raise your heels off the floor. Keep your shoulders pulled back and your head in a neutral position. Continue with your elbows fully extended and still pointing out.

Final Pull: With the barbell now touching the lower thigh, explosively extend your ankles, knees, and hips. Keep your shoulders over the bar, with the elbows fully extended as long as possible while the ankles, knees, and hips are extending. Shrug your shoulders and keep the arms fully extended during this time. Once the shoulders are completely elevated, flex your elbows quickly and pull your body under the bar by raising your arms as high as you can. The total accumulation of the upward acceleration will lift your feet off the floor.

Catch Phase: Once the bar reaches maximum height, rotate the bar with your arms and hands while pulling your body underneath the bar. At this time you will need to flex your ankles, knees, and hips into a half-squat position as your feet return to the floor slightly wider than when you started. The bar should be caught in line with the anterior deltoids.

Finish: Return the barbell to the floor by flexing your knees and hips and lowering the barbell to the thigh area. From here, continue to keep your back straight and lower the barbell by flexing your hips and knees, keeping the barbell close to your shins as you lower it to the floor.

Variations
You can perform this exercise using a kettle bell or a dumbbell with one arm at a time following the same procedures. The unbalanced nature of the single-arm variation recruits more of the core and shoulder stabilizers.

POWER CLEAN (continued)

Coaching Points This exercise is very complex and can be very dangerous. Begin learning the technique with a very light bar and no weights; you can even use a broomstick. Do not add weight to the movement until the technique is mastered.

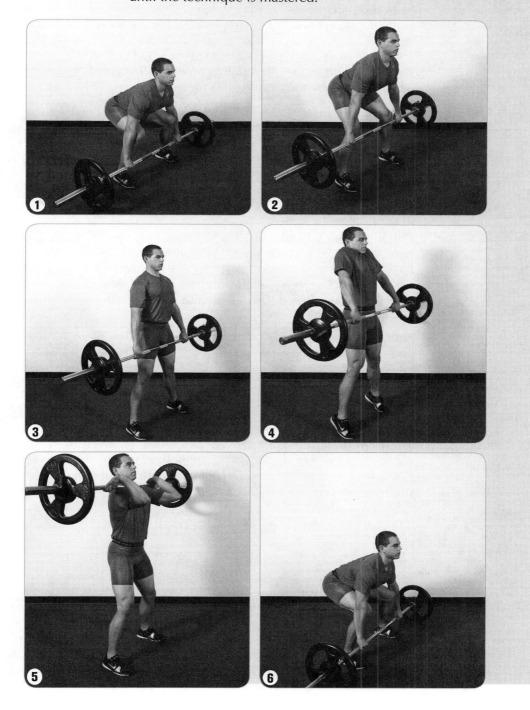

HANG CLEAN

Target	Glutes, quads, hamstrings, gastrocnemius and soleus, traps and delts
When	Early in the workout
Start	Hold the barbell with a pronated grip, your arms just outside of your thighs, and your arms extended. The barbell should be resting against your thighs. Keep your chest out, your shoulders back, and your head in a neutral position. Your feet should be just wider than shoulder-width apart with your toes pointing slightly out. Your body weight should be toward the balls of your feet.
Execution	**Pull Phase**: Explosively extend your ankles, knees, and hips. Keep your shoulders over the bar and elbows fully extended as long as possible while the ankles, knees, and hips are extending. Shrug your shoulders and keep the arms fully extended during this time. Once the shoulders are completely elevated, flex your elbows quickly and pull your body under the bar by raising your arms as high as you can. The total accumulation of the upward acceleration will lift your feet off the floor.
	Catch Phase: Once the bar reaches maximum height, rotate the bar with your arms and hands while pulling your body underneath the bar. At this point flex your ankles, knees, and hips into a half-squat position as your feet return to the floor slightly farther apart than when you started. The bar should be caught in line with the anterior deltoids.
	Finish: Return the barbell to the thigh area by flexing your knees and hips and extending your elbows.
Variations	You can perform this exercise using a dumbbell to work one arm at a time following the same procedures. The unbalanced nature of the single-arm variation recruits more of the core and shoulder stabilizers.
Coaching Points	This exercise is very complex and can be very dangerous. Begin learning the technique with a very light bar and no weights; you can even use a broomstick. Do not add weight to the movement until the technique is mastered.

HANG CLEAN *(continued)*

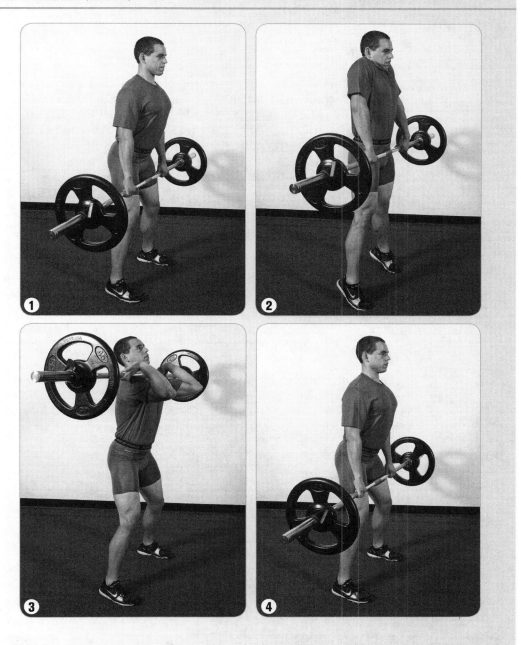

POWER SNATCH

Target   Glutes, quads, hamstrings, gastrocnemius and soleus, traps and delts

When   Early in the workout

Start   Stand with the balls of your feet under the bar and slightly wider than hip-width apart. Squat down and grip the bar with an overhand grip wider than shoulder-width apart (wider than the power clean grip). Your arms should be outside your knees and straight, with your elbows pointing out. Keep your head up (in a neutral position with the spine) with your chest out and shoulders pulled back. Position your shoulders over the bar with your back straight or slightly arched.

Execution   **Initial Pull**: Begin the power snatch by lifting the bar off the floor by extending your ankles, knees, and hips. (Make sure your hips and shoulders move at the same time and at the same pace). Keep your head in the neutral position with your back straight and arms fully extended as you pull the bar as close to your shins as you can.

Transition Phase: Drive your hips forward and move your body weight more toward the front of your feet, but do not raise your heels off the floor. Keep your shoulders pulled back and your head in a neutral position. Continue with your elbows fully extended and still pointing out.

Final Pull: With the barbell now touching the lower thigh, explosively extend your ankles, knees, and hips. Keep your shoulders over the bar while keeping the elbows fully extended as long as possible while the ankles, knees, and hips are extending. Shrug your

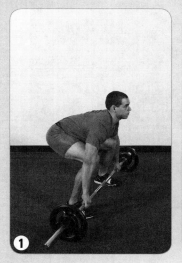

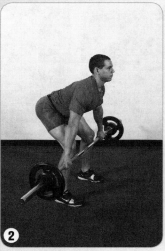

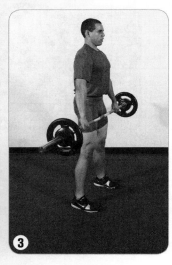

POWER SNATCH *(continued)*

shoulders and keep the arms fully extended during this time. Once the shoulders are completely elevated, flex your elbows quickly and pull your body under the bar by raising your arms as high as you can. The total accumulation of the upward acceleration will lift your feet off of the floor.

Catch Phase: Once the bar reaches maximum height, rotate the bar with your arms and hands while pulling your body underneath the bar. At this point flex your ankles, knees, and hips into a half-squat position as your feet return to the floor slightly wider than when you started. Extend your elbows to press the barbell up as your body moves down and under the bar. The bar is caught overhead with elbows extended, knees flexed, and your head in a neutral position. Stand upright with the bar directly over your head or slightly behind it.

Finish: Return the barbell to the floor by flexing your knees and hips and lowering the barbell to the thigh area. From here, continue to keep your back straight and lower the barbell by flexing your hips and knees, keeping the barbell close to your shins as you lower it to the floor.

Variations

You can perform this exercise using a dumbbell to work one arm at a time following the same procedures. The unbalanced nature of the single-arm variation recruits more of the core and shoulder stabilizers.

Coaching Points

This exercise is very complex and can be very dangerous. Begin learning the technique with a very light bar and no weights; you can even use a broomstick. Do not add weight to the movement until the technique is mastered.

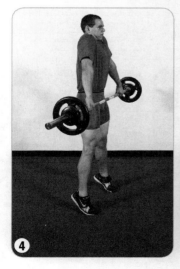
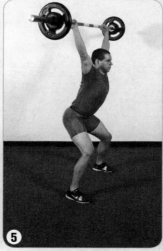
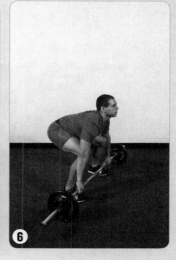

POWER JERK

Target
Glutes, quads, hamstrings, gastrocnemius and soleus, erector spinae, traps and delts

When
Early in the workout

Start
Hold a barbell at shoulder level with your hands slightly wider than shoulder-width apart, using a pronated grip. Keep your elbows up and in front of the barbell. Your head should be in a neutral position and your feet shoulder-width apart with your weight evenly distributed.

Execution
Drive Phase: Squat slightly (20 to 30 degrees) by flexing your ankles, knees, and hips. Make sure you keep your feet flat on the floor during the squat movement. Quickly reverse the direction of your body by extending your ankles, knees, and hips in an explosive manner. Drive upward with the lower body pushing the weight over your head. Focus on using your legs to drive the weight upward, not your arms. Your feet will leave the floor as you powerfully extend your entire body.

Lowering Phase: Slowly lower the barbell back to shoulder level in a controlled manner. If maximum weight is being attempted, dropping the barbell may be necessary. Only drop the weight if you are using bumper plates. Make sure you control the drop by not allowing the weight to bounce too high.

Variations
You can use split legs (one foot forward and one foot backward) during the drive as a variation of this exercise. The split position calls for more support from hip and ankle stabilizers.

Coaching Points
This exercise should be used with caution. If you cannot complete the lift, drop the barbell by pushing away from it and allowing it to fall. Do not try to hold on or catch the bar.

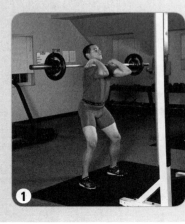 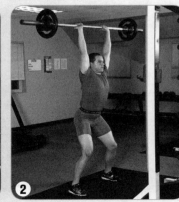 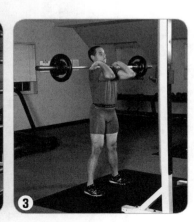

SQUAT JUMP

Target	Glutes, quads, hamstrings, gastrocnemius and soleus
When	End of the workout
Start	Stand with your feet just slightly wider than shoulder-width apart. Place your hands together and out in front of your upper body. Keep your back straight and your head in a neutral position.
Execution	Descend into a squat position by flexing your ankles, knees, and hips until your quads are parallel to the floor. Rapidly ascend by extending your ankles, knees, and hips explosively. This explosive movement will lift your body off the floor. Land softly by flexing your ankles, knees, and hips until you have returned to the squat position with your quads parallel to the floor.
Variations	You can also place your hands behind your head while performing this exercise. If you take the arm swing out of the exercise by placing your hands behind your head, you will increase the intensity of the exercise. After you have achieved proper strength and stability, you may use a weighted vest or light dumbbells for added resistance. Performing multiple continuous jumps places a greater demand on the muscles, giving them virtually no time to recover and adding an endurance component to the exercise.
Coaching Points	Practice landing softly. Never land with your knees locked. Make sure you keep your back straight, not rounded, especially during the landing phase.

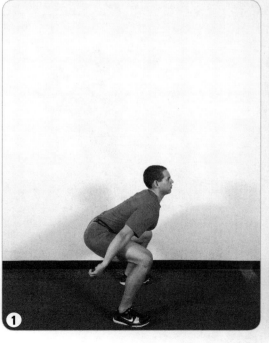

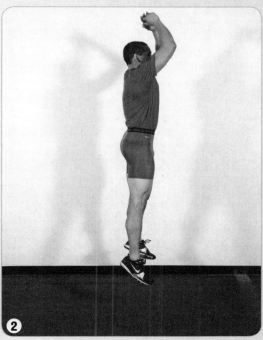

SPLIT SQUAT JUMP

Target   Glutes, quads, hamstrings, gastrocnemius and soleus

When   End of the workout

Start   Place feet in a split position with one foot in front of you and one foot behind you. Your feet should be far enough apart that you can create a 90-degree angle at your knee on the front leg. The back leg should be bent and your body weight split between the front foot and the back foot. Keep your torso upright with hands in front of your body.

Execution   Forcefully extend your ankles, knees, and hips in an upward movement. Both feet will come off the floor as your legs straighten. Land softly by flexing your ankles and knees, dispersing your weight evenly throughout both feet. Maintain an upright posture with your upper body.

Variations   Add light weight for extra resistance. You can also add a scissor kick (switching legs while you are in the air during the jump phase) to increase the difficulty of the movement and make the muscles work harder to maintain balance.

Coaching Points Make sure you do not collapse your upper body by flexing at the hips during the landing. You should maintain an upright posture throughout the exercise. You should also be sure to keep your feet far enough apart to maintain a 90-degree angle at the front knee.

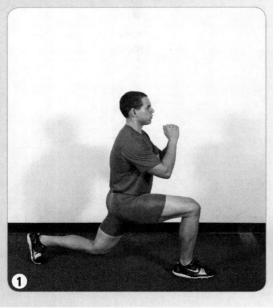

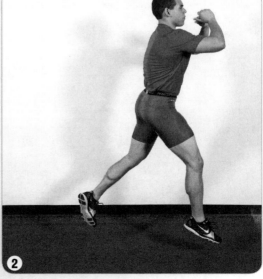

VERTICAL JUMP

Target	Glutes, quads, hamstrings, gastrocnemius and soleus
When	End of the workout
Start	Place your feet about shoulder-width apart. Flex your ankles, knees, and hips until your thighs are parallel to the floor. Keep the weight of your body on the balls of your feet.
Execution	Forcefully extend your ankles, knees, and hips in an upward movement. Swing your arms forward by flexing your shoulders. Both feet will come off the floor as your legs straighten. Land softly by flexing your ankles, and knees, dispersing your weight evenly throughout both feet. Maintain an upright posture with your upper body upon landing.
Variations	You can perform multiple vertical jumps in place to add a conditioning component to the exercise.
Coaching Points	Be sure the landing area is clear. Land softly with a slight bend in the knees and be careful not to collapse your upper body by flexing too far at the hips. Maintain a slight bend at the hips, but not so much that your chest reaches your thighs when landing. Land softly and do not lock your legs.

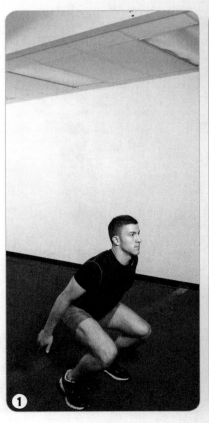
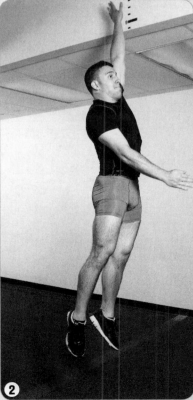

BROAD JUMP

Target	Glutes, quads, hamstrings, gastrocnemius and soleus
When	End of the workout
Start	Place your feet about shoulder-width apart. Flex your ankles, knees, and hips until your thighs are parallel to the floor. Keep the weight of your body on the balls of your feet.
Execution	Forcefully extend your ankles, knees, and hips in an upward and outward movement. Swing your arms forward by flexing your shoulders. Both feet will come off the floor as your legs straighten. Land softly by flexing your ankles and knees, dispersing your weight evenly throughout both feet. Maintain an upright posture with your upper body upon landing.
Variations	You can perform multiple broad jumps (3 or 4 reps) in a row to both add intensity to the exercise and increase the required power output.
Coaching Points	Do not collapse your upper body by flexing too much at the hips. Maintain a slight bend at the hips, but not so much that your chest reaches your thighs when landing. Be sure to land softly and do not lock your legs.

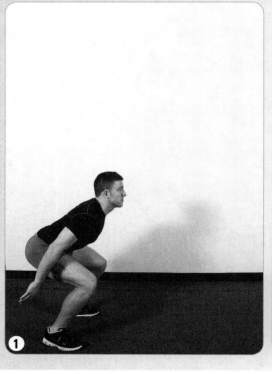
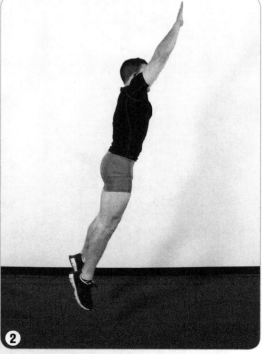

SINGLE-LEG TRIPLE JUMP

Target   Glutes, quads, hamstrings, gastrocnemius and soleus

When   End of the workout

Start   Stand on one leg with a slight bend in your knee and hip. Keep the weight of your body on the ball of your foot.

Execution   Forcefully extend your ankle, knee, and hip in an upward and outward movement. Swing your arms forward by flexing your shoulders. The foot of your working leg will come off the floor as your leg straightens. The nonworking leg will remain relaxed with a slight bend in the knee. Jump three times in a row and then land softly on both feet by flexing your ankles and knees, dispersing your weight evenly throughout both feet. Maintain an upright posture with your upper body upon landing.

Variations   You can perform this exercise but land on the same leg that you jump with. This will challenge the muscles of the nonworking leg by forcing them to help stabilize the body during the landing.

Coaching Points   Do not collapse your upper body by flexing too much at the hips when landing. Maintain a slight bend at the hips, but not so much that your chest reaches your thighs. Be sure to land softly and do not land with your legs locked out.

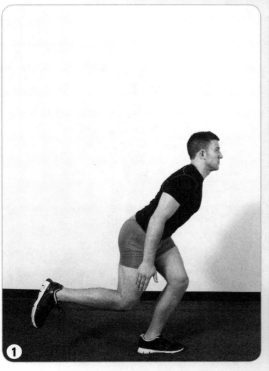

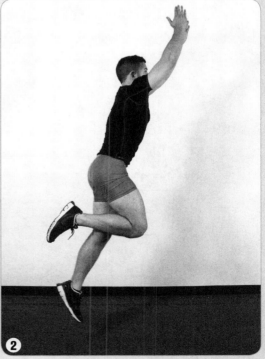

BENCH SINGLE-LEG BOUNDS

Target	Glutes, quads, hamstrings, gastrocnemius and soleus
When	End of the workout
Start	Stand with one foot on an exercise bench or a 12- to 16-inch stable box (30.5 to 40.6 cm). Stand upright with a slight bend in the knee of the leg that is still on the floor.
Execution	Forcefully extend your ankles, knees, and hips in an upward movement. Swing your arms forward by flexing your shoulders. Your involved foot (the one on the bench or box) will come off the bench as you jump. The uninvolved foot (the one on the floor) will also leave the floor as your leg straightens. Jump up and then land softly on the floor (with the uninvolved foot) and the bench (with the involved foot) at the same time. Maintain an upright posture with your upper body upon landing. Repeat the sequence quickly using the same leg for the prescribed number of repetitions.
Variations	You can perform this exercise alternating the legs during the jumps. This will add an element of balance and coordination.
Coaching Points	Do not collapse your upper body by flexing too much at the hips when landing. Maintain a slight bend at the hips, but not so much that your chest reaches your thighs. Be sure to land softly and do not lock your legs. Make sure you are using a very stable bench or box and that your landing area is clear of objects.

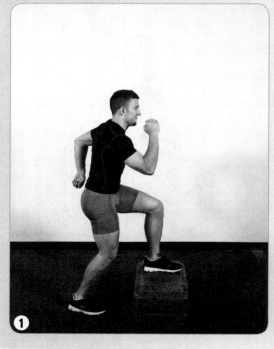

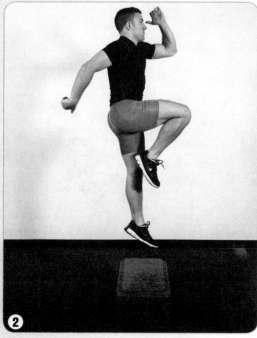

PART III

Goal-Oriented Lower-Body Workouts

CHAPTER 9

Increasing Mass and Strength

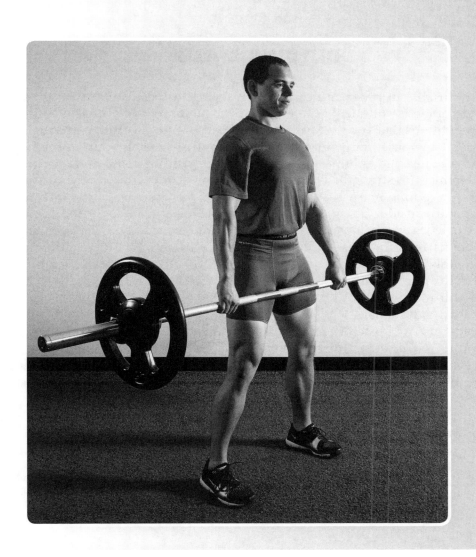

ecall from chapter 2 that intensity (how hard you train), duration (how long you train), frequency (how often you train), and volume (the number of exercises) determine the effectiveness of a training program. By manipulating these variables, you can work more specifically toward your individual goals. The two most common goals of training are increased size and greater strength. This chapter outlines ways to increase mass and strength in the legs and lower body and explains how to apply these gains to the activities you are most interested in.

Building bigger and stronger legs and lower body improves performance, intimidates competitors, and makes the body more aesthetically pleasing. Strength in the legs and lower body provides a solid base that is vital for most activities and sports. Strong legs support the knees, low back, and upper body.

BUILDING MASS

A key variable in program design when trying to increase muscle mass (hypertrophy) is volume. Volume is simply the number of exercises (sets) and repetitions that you perform per body part or muscle group. Although you can't increase your muscle mass without increasing your strength, you can adjust the volume to focus more on building mass and less on developing pure strength. The minimum number of exercises per muscle group for gaining mass is 4 to 6. For example, to add mass in the quads, you might consider doing front squats, single-leg squats, leg extensions, and single-leg extensions, all in the same exercise session. The optimal number of reps for mass building is 8 to 12. Performing 10 repetitions is probably ideal for mass building, doing 8 repetitions is leaning more toward the pure strength side (4 to 6 reps for strength), and doing 12 reps takes you more toward the muscular endurance side (14 to 16 reps for muscular endurance).

Rest is also a big factor in mass-building programs. As with repetitions, the preferred number for mass-building rest periods falls somewhere between those for pure strength (up to 5 minutes) and muscular endurance (20 to 45 seconds). For mass building, a rest period of 60 to 90 seconds is ideal. Finally, the load (the amount of weight you are lifting) should be in the moderate to heavy range. You do not want to lift max or near-max loads, but the load must be challenging enough to exhaust the muscle.

UNILATERAL TRAINING
FOR BALANCED STRENGTH

Lower-body unilateral strength movements focus on one leg moving independently of the other, while bilateral lower-body strength movements are those exercises that use both legs at the same time. The barbell squat and the leg press are two good examples of bilateral lower-body exercises. Both of these movements are generally performed with both legs at the same time. It would be very difficult to perform a barbell squat with one leg. Balancing the bar with the weight plates on the sides would be almost impossible and very dangerous. A leg press can be done with one leg; however, most leg-press machines are designed for the user to press with both legs.

Unilateral lower-body exercises, on the other hand, work each leg independently; lunges and step-ups are examples of such exercises. A lunge exercise primarily works the leg that steps forward, while the rear leg is used for balance and stability. The same thing applies for a step-up exercise. The leg on the bench or box does the majority of the work while the opposite leg is used for stability and balance.

Most body-weight exercises can be done unilaterally and performed virtually anywhere with little or no equipment. These exercises are important for gaining strength in muscle groups that are not properly balanced, and they also help with overall body awareness, balance, and coordination. Unilateral strength training is a good way to add variety to your workouts while helping to prevent injury.

Imbalances in certain muscles or muscle groups may develop naturally. For example, the quads are naturally bigger and stronger than the hamstrings because they are designed to bear more weight. Although this type of imbalance is normal, it is important not to exacerbate it with quad-heavy training. Some athletes are naturally dominant on one side; again the goal is not to exacerbate the imbalance. Imbalances arise in other ways. Working one part of the body heavily and neglecting another can create a muscle imbalance. Athletes often develop muscle imbalance while training and competing: Baseball players and golfers forcefully rotate (swing) in one direction over and over; place kickers and punters repeatedly kick with the same leg; tennis, racquetball, and squash players swing with the same arm and drive off the same leg. Muscle imbalance can also occur when an injury is not properly rehabilitated and recovery is incomplete. Nerve damage and atrophy (weakness and shrinkage of the muscle) can then perpetuate the imbalance. These scenarios make it very important for athletes to have well-rounded weight-training programs as well as proper injury prevention and rehabilitation strategies.

Regardless of the reason for the unbalanced strength development, you should design your program to develop balanced strength, both from front to back and from right to left. Bilateral exercises typically do not allow you to balance your strength gains as well as unilateral exercises do. For example, if you have a weakness in one leg due to an old injury, when you squat with a barbell this leg will do less work than the stronger leg. Over time, the stronger leg will carry more of the work load and continue to get stronger while the weaker leg simply goes along for the ride and gets weaker and weaker. This weakness can also lead to incorrect posture and mechanics, which in turn can lead to injuries in other parts of the body. Conversely, a unilateral exercise, like a lunge, will allow each leg to work independently of one another and even out any strength imbalances. Unlike the barbell squat, the lunge exercise will allow the weaker leg to catch up to the stronger leg by placing greater demand on it.

STRENGTH TRAINING FOR SPORT

When you are strength training for sports, consider a few key points. First, unlike traditional strength-training routines, training programs for sport performance must be designed around distinct periods, each with its own goals and objectives. This training method, called periodization, is crucial to a successful strength-training program for sport performance. Athletes in many sports, such as soccer and ice hockey, have distinct seasons, and their programs must be designed around their particular sport seasons. The typical periods of this type of program design are preseason (preparation phase), in-season (maintenance phase), and off-season (recovery phase).

The preseason is the time to get your body ready for a long, demanding season. Many sports have seasons that can last 3 to 10 months depending on your level of play. The start of the preseason training period should consist of a basic strength-training program (1 or 2 sets of 10 to 12 reps with moderate loads) followed by a hypertrophy phase (3 or 4 sets of 8 to 10 reps with moderate to heavy loads). Depending on your sport, a period of strength and power training (3 or 4 sets of 4 to 6 reps with heavy loads) would follow your hypertrophy phase.

The in-season period is a time to maintain what you have worked so hard for in the preseason (1 or 2 sets of 6 to 8 reps with moderate to heavy loads). Again, many sport seasons are several months long, and a detraining effect with a loss of strength will occur if you do not maintain some kind of resistance program during the competitive season.

The purpose of the off-season period is twofold. First, the off-season allows for physical and mental recovery from a long, competitive season. The pressure of competition and the daily grind of sport participation can lead to burnout and mental fatigue. The off-season is a great time to recharge your batteries by getting away from the sport. At this time you should address any injuries that may have occurred during the season. Physical therapy may be necessary at this point for addressing any injuries that may not have healed on their own. Second, the end of the off-season period serves as the transition to, or the beginning of, the preseason period. This is the time to begin a light training period to get your body ready for the more intense work that is about to come in the second half of the preseason.

From here the cycle begins all over again. The length of each phase will depend on the length of your season, your sport, and your specific goals. The goal of this periodization model is to reach peak performance levels at the start of the season, to maintain this high level as long as possible throughout the season while reducing the chances of injury, and to refresh and recover before returning to intense training.

STRENGTH TRAINING FOR ENDURANCE ACTIVITIES

Strength training for endurance athletes has been controversial. Many endurance athletes and trainers think that there is no place for developing strength in an endurance training program. While it is true that endurance activities, such as marathon running, rely mostly on repetitive aerobic movements, closer examination suggests there is probably room for developing and maintaining strength in preparation for endurance sports. Endurance activities such as long-distance running, long-distance swimming, and triathlons call on mostly slow-twitch muscle fibers for movement and use aerobic energy systems as their main sources of fuel. Strength and power activities such as softball, sprinting, and golf call on mostly fast-twitch muscle fibers for movement and use anaerobic energy systems for their main sources of fuel. However, when an exercise activity is performed, the body never uses just one type of muscle fiber group or one energy system.

The body goes through stages of recruitment of muscle fiber types in accordance with the demands placed on them. The same thing applies with the energy systems. The middle of a marathon will be fueled mostly by aerobic energy, but the sprint at the end will be fueled mostly by anaerobic energy systems. Therefore, it makes sense that, when designing endurance-related training programs, you should include strength- and power-related movements. For example, stronger muscles in the core and upper body may help a marathon runner maintain posture and proper mechanics, allowing the runner to be more efficient. This increased efficiency may spare energy that can be used to finish the event faster. Furthermore, even the longest endurance activities usually involve a sprint at some point in the event. Hill climbing (often required in biking and running) also requires spurts of strength and power. Pushing off the side of the pool during flip turns or sprinting across the finish line in a rowing event require strength and power that can be increased by a good strength-training program. In addition, all endurance sports require repetitive motions that may create muscle imbalances. Strength training helps you overcome these muscle imbalances that can lead to injury. Finally, strength training can assist in overall wellness by slowing the loss of muscle mass and increasing bone density, both of which are associated with aging. (Swimmers especially are prone to a loss in bone density because the sport isn't a weight-bearing activity.)

MULTIPLANAR TRAINING

Most traditional leg-strengthening programs are segmented into working the quads, hamstrings, and calves. Some programs may include the glutes as well. This body-part-training approach only scratches the surface of true strength development, especially when it comes to the legs. Exercises such as the leg curl, leg extension, and calf raise work with movements at only one joint and in one plane. We would consider these exercises uniplanar joint movements. These exercises are great for aesthetics and for certain phases of rehabilitation programs. The problem with such movement patterns is there is really no functionality to them. In other words, they do not mirror more complex movements that you make every day, especially while performing full- or nearly full-body activities and participating in sports. Movements in one plane do very little to stimulate motor memory; therefore, they do not improve your ability to move in multiple planes simultaneously.

The human body moves in three planes, and specific types of movements occur in each plane. The sagittal plane divides the body into left and right halves, and the movements that take place within it go forward and backward (as well as up and down). An example of a lower-body exercise in the sagittal plane is the leg extension.

The frontal, or coronal, plane divides the body into front and back halves, and the movements that occur within it are side-to-side motions. Abduction movements (away from the midline) and adduction movements (toward the midline) are examples of lower-body movements in the frontal plane. Both can be performed with free weights or machines.

The transverse plane divides the body into top and bottom halves, and the movements that take place within it are mostly rotational. The walking lunge with rotation is a good example of an exercise in the transverse plane.

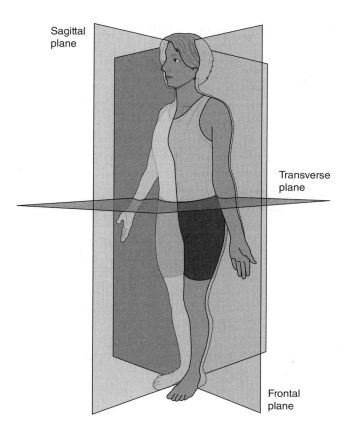

Sagittal plane

Transverse plane

Frontal plane

Because the legs and torso are connected by the hips, you must use closed-chain multiplanar exercises (explained later in this chapter), such as the multidirectional lunge and the lateral step-up, to develop a strong foundation for total-body strength. The great range of motion at the hip joint (flexion, extension, abduction, adduction, internal rotation, and external rotation) makes multiplanar exercises a necessity in a well-rounded program. Multiplanar movements are a great way to develop strong, functional legs. Whether you're a football running back who needs to make quick cuts and drive opponents forward, a competitive weightlifter who wants strength *and* size, a construction worker who moves heavy materials from one place to another, or a parent who hoists a young child in and out of the car seat, tub, and bed, multiplanar exercises can help you move more freely and effectively and reduce your chance of injury. Developing strength through multiple planes helps build speed and agility for athletics as well as greater stability and ease of movement for everyday activities.

FUNCTIONAL TRAINING

Functional lower-body training refers to exercises that increase strength and stability in the legs and lower body using movements that mimic those performed in everyday life. Functional exercises will ultimately allow you to perform daily activities with more efficiency and less chance of injury. Climbing stairs, picking up or playing with your children, lifting household items, and performing hobbies and sports are all examples of everyday activities that will be enhanced by performing functional leg exercises.

Most functional leg exercises are what are termed closed-chain exercises. Closed-chain exercises are those in which the distal end of an extremity (usually the hand or foot) is in a fixed position during an exercise. (In open-chain exercises, the distal end is not fixed in place.) In other words, in a closed-chain exercise, the hand or foot remains in contact with the floor or the platform of a machine. Closed-chain exercises are usually weight bearing and involve multiple joints, such as the lunge and the squat. Because of this, they are considered more functional (mimicking real-life movements) and are therefore used more often by athletes when training for sports. They are also used during more aggressive stages of physical rehabilitation. Inactivity from surgery, being on crutches, or overcompensation due to injury may lead to disruption of the body's normal movement patterns. These movement patterns must be relearned through various forms of functional training.

Functional leg exercises promote coordination through multiple movement patterns performed in synchronicity. This coordinated movement leads to the development of new neural pathways, commonly referred to as muscle memory. Body-weight squatting, lunging patterns, and single-leg deadlifts are examples of functional training exercises that assist with the relearning of normal movement patterns after an injury.

Open-chain exercises are those movements in which the hand (upper-body exercises) or the foot (lower-body exercises) is free to move, and these exercises are usually non-weight bearing. Open-chain movements usually involve movements at the elbow for the upper body (biceps curls) or at the knee for the lower body (knee extensions). Open-chain exercises are great for isolating muscles and muscle groups and are appropriate for earlier stages of rehabilitation and bodybuilding. For example, the leg-extension machine isolates the quad muscles on the front of the thigh, but it does very little to increase stability in the knee during movement activities such as sprinting, jumping, and changes of direction. Open-chain exercises will do very little for improving stability and mobility around a joint or series of joints. Therefore, you should use open-chain exercises sparingly for sport performance training and the later stages of injury rehabilitation.

CHAPTER 10

Boosting Power and Stamina

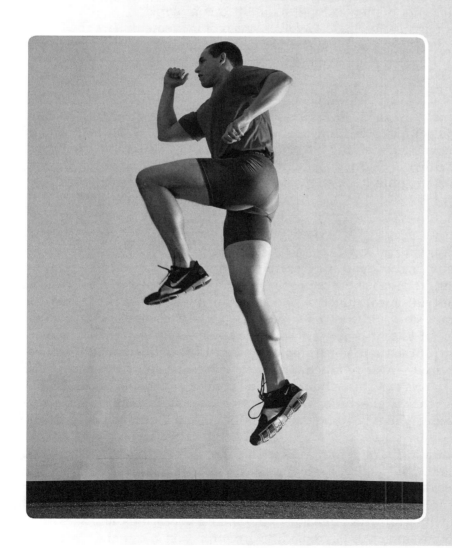

One way to think of strength is as the ability to generate as much force as possible during one repetition. The standard measurement of strength is the 1-repetition maximum, known as 1RM. If we were to put this in the form of an equation, the formula for strength would look like this:

$$\text{Strength} = \text{mass} \times \text{distance}$$

In other words, strength is measured in terms of moving an object of a given mass over a certain distance. You may notice that there is no concept for time in this equation. It doesn't matter how long it takes you to complete the task, only that it gets completed. Good examples of pure strength exercises are the maximum squat and the bench press. When strength is being assessed, even in competition, the speed a heavy load is moved does not matter, as long as the lift is completed.

Power, on the other hand, involves speed of movement; here the length of time involved to complete the task is very important. If we were to put power in the form of an equation it would look like this:

$$\text{Power} = \text{work} \div \text{time}$$

Power is often referred to as speed-strength. Unlike strength, the time it takes to complete the movement is very important. Good examples of power movements are the power clean and the vertical jump. You can't perform either of these movements slowly. This chapter looks at ways to tailor your program to develop power and endurance, or stamina.

BUILDING POWER

Most traditional weightlifting exercises can be done at varying tempos. Increasing the speed of the return of a lift will work on power development. Take the squat, for instance. A good rule for the beginner is to lower the weight in a slow and controlled manner (about 2 seconds), take a slight pause (about 1 second) at the bottom, and then return to the starting position in about the same time it took to lower the weight (about 2 seconds). For increased power production, the tempo would be much faster. The lowering phase can still remain slow and controlled (about 2 seconds), but as soon as the weight reaches the bottom of the lift, it should be returned immediately. There is no hold at the bottom, and the return is as fast as possible.

In addition to performing traditional lifts with a fast tempo, if you are interested in increasing your power production, you should include two types of power exercises in your program. The first group of power-developing exercises is the Olympic lifts. These exercises use speed and strength with a forceful extension of the ankles, knees, hips, and back. Two very good examples of Olympic lifts are the power clean and the power snatch (see chapter 8 for detailed descriptions). These exercises must be done at maximum speed, and their performance is very technical. Since these exercises involve virtually the entire body, they are excellent for overall strength gains as well as power production. The intensity and full range of motion required for executing these lifts also assist with calorie burn and flexibility.

The second category of power exercises is plyometrics. Plyometric exercises are movements that train muscles to reach maximum strength in the shortest possible time. These types of exercises include jumping in place, bounding, and doing box hops. Athletes who want to increase their first-step quickness, vertical jump, and overall power for their sports use plyometric exercises. Plyometric exercises, along with the development of eccentric strength through closed-chain exercises, are critical for preventing injury as well as returning to play after injury in the lower body, especially the knee.

POWER TRAINING FOR ENDURANCE

Recall from chapter 9 that increases in strength may benefit long-distance runners, bikers, and swimmers by sparing energy expenditure, increasing the ability to maintain proper mechanics, reducing injury, and assisting with strong sprint finishes and hill climbs. Power workouts also help in these areas. In fact, the benefits derived from power training may even be more substantial than the benefits from strength training alone. Plyometric exercises, which are a great way to increase power, may actually help endurance runners decrease foot contact time on the ground. The decreased time the foot is on the ground would increase performance, specifically speed, especially over the course of a very long race. Even a small improvement over the course of an event that is a couple of hours long could potentially add up to several minutes saved on overall time.

Power-endurance training (power stamina) is very important for sports such as wrestling. Unlike running or biking, wrestling requires constant use of muscular strength throughout a match. This taxes the anaerobic energy system for prolonged periods. The high-intensity, maximal-effort movements need to be reproduced over and over again. Power stamina is the key to success in activities that require repeated high-intensity movements. You can increase power endurance by performing supersets with very little or no rest between exercises. However, I do want to be very clear: Plyometric training is anaerobic in nature. This type of training calls on the creatine phosphate system for maximum energy storage resulting in maximum power output. If full recovery (up to 1 minute) between sets is not allowed, you will not see the full benefits of power training. Plyometric training should never be used for conditioning or aerobic training.

Proper recovery time is necessary for full energy restoration, resulting in greater energy expenditure for the next set. The quality of the movement versus the quantity of the movement should always be stressed. You will see much better results and reduce your chance for injury if you follow these guidelines.

COMPLEX TRAINING

It is clear that strength and power exercises can actually help endurance athletes maintain proper mechanics; develop stronger, more powerful sprints; and reduce overuse injuries. Power workouts, more specifically plyometrics, can help runners decrease foot contact time and assist with training the creatine phosphate system, allowing the body to reach its maximum power output. Strength and power training come together in the form of complex training.

Complex training calls for a high-intensity strength exercise followed by a plyometric exercise, with prescribed rest periods between the pairs of exercises as well as between the exercises themselves. Because of the high-intensity workloads followed by periods of rest, complex training can be used as a form of interval training. Interval training is a great way to increase overall endurance for sports or everyday activities. It can increase anaerobic metabolism as well as increase oxygen consumption. The prescribed rest periods during interval training allow you to perform a greater amount of overall work than you would with steady exercise. Complex training shares this feature. By pairing a strength movement with a plyometric exercise, with very little rest in between, the body will learn to adapt to greater overall volumes of work at higher intensities. Complex training may enhance your overall endurance when you add it to a periodized training program. Increased endurance is a must not only for endurance athletes but also for those who want to enhance their quality of life. You can increase strength by using complex training, but just as important, the increase in stamina from complex training will allow you to train harder during your normal strength-training sessions, resulting in greater strength gains. You can add complex training to a strength-training program to increase cardiorespiratory endurance, muscular endurance, and power.

Complex training is an advanced form of exercise that will increase your workload capacity and power output in a short time. Simply stated, complex training involves pairing a high-intensity strength exercise (a squat for example) with an explosive plyometric type of exercise (a squat jump for example) with very little rest between sets. To truly understand it, we must take a closer look into the physiology of the muscular and nervous systems.

Our bodies contain two types of muscle fibers, fast-twitch and slow-twitch fibers. The slow-twitch (type I) fibers produce submaximal force over longer periods. Most aerobic activities, such as long-distance running, call on slow-twitch muscle fibers for their work production. The fast-twitch (type IIa and type IIb) fibers produce maximal forces for shorter periods. Power activities, such as sprinting and hitting a baseball, call on type II muscle fibers for their work production.

The nervous system tells the muscular system what fibers to recruit and when to recruit them. Neurons dictate which fibers (fast-twitch or slow-twitch) are needed for a particular movement. As Don Chu notes in his book *Explosive Power and Strength* (Human Kinetics, 1996), specific training methods, such as complex training, that improve motoneuron recruitment may actually teach slow-twitch muscle fibers to act more like fast-twitch muscle fibers. Highly trained athletes get the most out of their training by efficiently recruiting fast-twitch muscle fibers as well as encouraging the slow-twitch fibers to act more like fast-twitch fibers. The strength exercise used in the first half of complex training will fire up, or excite, the motor neurons, and the plyometric exercise in the second half will take advantage of this excited period and train the body's nervous system to work more efficiently. The length of the rests within the pairings (the time between the strength exercise and the plyometric exercise) and between the pairings (the length of the rest between each strength–plyometric pair) will vary based on your particular goals and fitness level.

Generally, if you are just beginning to train, you should rest from 30 seconds to 90 seconds *within* the pairs of exercises and 1 to 3 minutes *between* the pairs of exercises. More advanced people may rest from 1 to 3 minutes within the pairs of exercises and 3 to 5 minutes between the pairs of exercises. Adding complex training to your workouts is a great way to shock your body into producing gains. By varying the workouts, you have a smaller chance of adapting and a greater chance of increasing speed, power, and strength. Complex training is also an excellent way to break through training plateaus; the intensity and novelty of these movement combinations allow you to work through lulls in your training program. Complex training also provides a very intense workout in a short time.

CHAPTER **11**

Ready-Made
Workouts

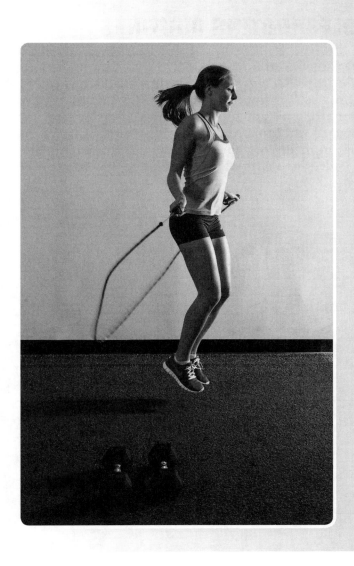

The following are common programs that may be used for various situations, such as when you are trying to develop strength, size, or endurance in a specific muscle or muscle group, or when time is short. You can use these ready-made workouts instead of your current program, or in addition to your current program, as a means of mixing things up. Feel free to make substitutions for specific exercises if you have an injury or if you simply do not like a particular movement. Use the specified number of sets and reps for each exercise as a guideline rather than an absolute prescription. Make sure you are warmed up properly before going into these routines. Do 1 or 2 sets of the first exercise in each program as a warm-up to make sure you are ready to dive right in at a fairly high intensity.

TROUBLESHOOTING ROUTINES

Everyone has weak areas that need improvement. These troubleshooting routines address specific problem areas such as small quads, skinny calves, and flat glutes. You will also find routines that save time, allow you to work on cardiorespiratory training, and focus on strength development. By reviewing chapters 2 and 3, you can also design your own routines using these general guidelines to meet your specific goals. With the templates provided, along with your personal designs, the variations that can be created are almost endless.

BODY-WEIGHT LEG STRENGTHENER

Explanation   Body-weight exercises build functional strength, stability, and balance. They also use very little or no equipment, making them ideal if you travel often or have limited access to equipment.

Muscles Worked   Glutes, quads, hamstrings

Variations   Add intensity to the routine by holding a dumbbell, weight plate, medicine ball, or any other weighted implement. Decrease the rest period between sets to 30 seconds to 1 minute for an added challenge.

Exercise	Sets	Reps
Squat	3	10-12
Wide squat	3	10-12
Split squat	2	10
Single-leg toe touch	2	10
Single-leg squat	2	8-10
Rest between sets: 1 to 2 minutes.		

MACHINE-BASED LEG STRENGTHENER

Explanation   Machine-based exercises are a safe, effective way to build bigger, stronger legs. Machine-based programs are great for beginners, but they can also be very useful for advanced weight trainers.

Muscles Worked   Quads, glutes, hamstrings, calves

Variations   You can substitute similar machines for many of the exercises in this routine. For instance, a leg sled may be substituted for the 45-degree leg-press machine, and a seated leg-curl machine may be substituted for the supine leg-curl machine.

Exercise	Sets	Reps
Smith press squat	4	10, 8, 6, 4
Leg press	3	8-10
Leg extension	3	8-10
Leg curl	3	8-10
Machine standing calf raise	3	8-10
Machine seated calf raise	3	8-10
Rest between sets: 1 to 2 minutes.		

FREE-WEIGHT MUSCLE-BALANCE BUILDER

Explanation   Free weights are ideal for advanced lifters and athletes because of the stability and balance involved during their execution. Free-weight routines are also great for creating muscle balance in the lower body.

Muscles Worked   Quads, glutes, hamstrings, low back, calves

Variations   Beginning lifters should start with 1 or 2 sets of each exercise and work up to the 2 to 4 sets that are prescribed.

Muscle group or region targeted	Exercise	Sets	Reps
Glutes and quads	Barbell or dumbbell squat	4	10, 8, 6, 4
Glutes and quads	Step-up	3	8-10
Glutes and quads	Walking lunge	3	8-10
Hamstrings, glutes, and calves	Romanian deadlift	3	8-10
Glutes and hamstrings	Ankle-weight hip extension	2	8-10
Soleus	Seated calf raise	2	8-10
Gastrocnemius	Standing calf raise	2	8-10
Rest between sets: 1 to 2 minutes.			

EXERCISE-BALL WORKOUT

Explanation   The only equipment needed for this routine is an exercise ball. The instability created by the ball makes it a great routine for working on balance and core stabilization as well as leg strength.

Muscles Worked   Glutes, hamstrings, low back, quads, calves

Variations   You can perform the leg curl, bridging, and squat exercises with a single leg. The single-leg versions of these exercises are very difficult and will make the routine very intense, both on the involved muscles and the surrounding stabilizing muscles. If you perform these exercises using a single leg, you will double the time it takes to complete this routine.

Muscle group or region targeted	Exercise	Sets	Reps
Glutes, hamstrings, and low back	Exercise-ball lying hip extension	2	12
Glutes and quads	Exercise-ball squat	2	12
Glutes and hamstrings	Double-leg bridge on exercise ball	2	12
Hamstrings and glutes	Exercise-ball leg curl	2*	12
*Go to the top and repeat the sequence.			
Rest 10 to 20 seconds between exercises if needed.			

QUAD DEVELOPER

Explanation   To develop huge quads, you will need to work with a high volume of sets and reps. A mixture of machines and free weights will also challenge your quads to grow.

Muscles Worked   Quads, glutes, calves

Variations   If a sled is not available, you can do the walking lunge without it. If you have trouble performing the front squat because of shoulder tightness or injury, do a back squat instead.

Exercise	Sets	Reps
Front squat	3-4	10-12
Weighted-sled walking lunge	3	10-15 yards
Exercise-ball squat	3	10-12
Single-leg squat	3	10
Machine leg extension	3-4	10-12
Single-leg extension	3	10-12
Rest between sets: 1 to 2 minutes.		

HAMSTRING DEVELOPER

Explanation   Work the hamstring group with machines and free weights in order to develop them in a strong yet functional manner.

Muscles Worked   Hamstrings, glutes, low back

Variations   Romanian deadlifts may be substituted for straight-leg deadlifts if you have back discomfort.

Exercise	Sets	Reps
Straight-leg deadlift	3	8-10
Single-leg toe touch	3	8-10
Prone leg curl	3	8-10
Hamstring lower	2	6-8
Exercise-ball supine leg curl	2	10-12
Rest between sets: 1 to 2 minutes.		

CALF DEVELOPER

Explanation Developing big calves is probably one of the hardest things to do in weight training. Be patient and consistent with this routine to reach your goal.

Muscles Worked Calves (gastrocnemius and soleus)

Variations Feel free to change your foot placement on the floor or the platform of the machine during these exercises; a slight turn inward or outward will slightly change the way the muscle is worked. Consider performing 1 set with your feet straight ahead, 1 set with your feet turned slightly inward, and 1 set with your feet turned slightly outward.

Exercise	Sets	Reps
Machine standing calf raise	3-4	10-12
Standing calf raise	3	10-12
Machine seated calf raise	3-4	10-12
Seated calf raise	3	10-12
Functional-trainer standing calf raise	3	10-12
Rest between sets: 1 to 2 minutes.		

MULTIJOINT WORKOUT

Explanation This routine increases strength and explosive power at the same time. Because of the intensity of these exercises, the rest period between sets is longer than for most of the other workouts.

Muscles Worked Quads, glutes, hamstrings, calves

Variations You can substitute the hang clean for the power clean, and you can substitute the broad jump for the vertical jump. These substitutions will add variety to the workout.

Exercise	Sets	Reps
Power clean	2-3	10
Power snatch	2-3	10
Vertical jump	3	8-10
Single-leg triple jump	2 each leg	6-8
Rest 1 to 3 minutes between sets.		

MUSCULAR-ENDURANCE AND HEART-PUMPING ROUTINES

Weight training is most often used to increase size and strength. However, it can also be used to increase muscular endurance and calorie burn and therefore increase fat loss. In these heart-pumping routines, the reps will be much higher (10 to 20) than in the strength and size routines, and the rest periods will be much shorter (5 to 30 seconds) than in the size and strength routines as well. Keeping the heart rate elevated is the key to burning more calories and fat; therefore compound exercises are a very important part of these routines. Compound exercises will use more muscles and muscle groups and thus use more energy. The following routines may be more intense than what you are used to. Make sure you ease your way into these routines slowly by beginning with 1 or 2 sets of each exercise and then working your way up to 3 sets. Circuit training and superset exercises with very little rest will keep your pace fast and intensity high, resulting in a heart-pumping routine.

BODY-WEIGHT CIRCUIT

Explanation   The body-weight circuit can be done virtually anywhere with very little or no equipment. This circuit is ideal if you are traveling or in a hurry, or if you do not have access to equipment. Perform 1 set of each exercise in the prescribed order. Repeat the sequence to the number of sets listed.

Muscles Worked   Quads, glutes, calves

Variations   Add jump rope work (skipping 20 to 30 times) or a 6-inch box (15 cm) step-up set (20 to 30 steps rapidly up and down) between exercises for increased heart-pumping intensity.

Muscle group or region targeted	Exercise	Sets	Reps
Glutes and quads	Body-weight squat	3	12-15
Glutes and quads	Squat jump	3	8-10
Quads, glutes, and hamstrings	Split squat	3	12-15
Quads, glutes, and hamstrings	Split squat jump	3	6-8
Quads, glutes, and hamstrings	Walking lunge	3	10-15 yards
Rest between sets only as needed to maintain form. Rest between circuits: 1 to 2 minutes.			

MACHINE CIRCUIT

Explanation   Most health clubs devote an area of the gym to selectorized equipment. In fact, many place these machines in a circuit format, allowing users to move quickly from machine to machine. Machine circuits are a great way to mix up your normal free-weight routine. Perform 1 set of each exercise in the prescribed order. Repeat the sequence to reach the number of sets listed.

Muscles Worked   Quads, hamstrings, glutes, calves

Variations   You can reduce the rest period between circuits to less than the prescribed 1 to 2 minutes if your fitness level allows. Raise the reps to 15 to 20 once the 12 to 15 range becomes too easy.

Muscle group or region targeted	Exercise	Sets	Reps
Glutes and quads	Smith press squat	3	12-15
Hamstrings	Leg curl	3	12-15
Quads and glutes	Leg press	3	12-15
Quads	Leg extension	3	12-15
Gastrocnemius	Standing calf raise	3	12-15
Rest between sets only as needed to maintain form. Rest between circuits: 1 to 2 minutes.			

FREE-WEIGHT CIRCUIT

Explanation The free-weight circuit is easy to do with very little equipment. It is ideal for small spaces or if you have no machines available. Perform 1 set of each exercise in the prescribed order. Repeat the sequence to the number of sets listed.

Muscles Worked Quads, glutes, hamstrings, calves

Variations Wear a weighted vest while performing this routine to increase the intensity.

Muscle group or region targeted	Exercise	Sets	Reps
Glutes and quads	Dumbbell squat	3	12-15
Glutes and quads	Step-up	3	12-15
Glutes and quads	Single-leg bench squat	3	12-15
Hamstrings, glutes, and calves	Romanian deadlift	3	12-15
Quads and glutes	Step-down	3	12-15
Rest between sets only as needed to maintain form. Rest between circuits: 1 to 2 minutes.			

SUPERSET UNILATERAL WORKOUT

Explanation   Superset workouts are great for increasing the heart rate and limiting the time taken to complete a routine. The pairings of the exercises will help build in rest time for the opposing muscle group as well as create balance in muscle development.

Muscles Worked   Quads, glutes, hamstrings, lower legs, hip flexors, low back

Variations   You may substitute other unilateral exercises in this routine. Just be sure that you choose exercises that work opposing muscles or muscle groups (e.g., quads vs. hamstrings).

Muscle group or region targeted	Exercise	Sets	Reps
Glutes and quads	Single-leg press	3	12, 10, 8
Hamstrings, glutes, and calves	Single-leg Romanian deadlift	3	12, 10, 8
Glutes and quads	Step-up	3	12, 10, 8
Glutes and hamstrings	Single-leg bridge	3	8-10
Quads	Single-leg extension	3	12, 10, 8
Hamstrings	Single-leg curl	3	12, 10, 8
Gastrocnemius	Single-leg calf raise	3	12, 10, 8
Tibialis anterior	Heel walk	3	10-15 yards
Hip flexors and quads	4-way hip-machine flexion	3	12, 10, 8
Glutes and hamstrings	4-way hip-machine extension	3	12, 10, 8
Rest between exercises only as needed to maintain form. Rest between supersets: 1 to 2 minutes.			

TIME-SAVING ROUTINES

In the real world, you do not always have an hour or more to complete your workout. Work, family, and other obligations often cut into your available time. As is the case with all exercise, even a shorter workout is better than no workout at all. The following routines take advantage of circuits and supersets to speed up the time required to complete them. When time is of the essence, pick one of these routines to keep you on track. You don't necessarily have to miss a workout even when your life pulls you in many directions.

30-MINUTE LEG STRENGTHENER

Explanation   Perform these exercises in order. They are arranged to provide some recovery time to the muscle group that is not being worked. This should allow you to get through each muscle group three times with very little rest.

Muscles Worked   Quads, hamstrings, glutes, lower leg

Variations   Substitute virtually any other quad, hamstring, glute, or lower-leg exercise from part II of this book into this routine to add variety.

Muscle group or region targeted	Exercise	Sets	Reps
Quads	Exercise-ball squat	1	10
Hamstrings	Straight-leg deadlift	1	10
Glutes	Walking lunge	1	15 yards
Lower leg	Machine standing calf raise	1	10
Quads	Split squat	1	8
Hamstrings	Exercise-ball supine leg curl	1	10
Glutes	Step-up	1	10
Lower leg	Machine seated calf raise	1	10
Quads	Walking retro lunge	1	15 yards
Hamstrings	Prone leg curl	1	10
Glutes	Leg press	1	10
Lower leg	Standing calf raise	1	10
Rest between exercises only as needed to maintain proper form.			

20-MINUTE LEG STRENGTHENER

Explanation   Perform these exercises in order. They are arranged to provide some recovery time to the muscle group that is not being worked. This should allow you to get through each muscle group three times with very little rest.

Muscles Worked   Quads, hamstrings, glutes, lower leg

Variations   Substitute virtually any other quad, hamstring, glute, or lower-leg exercise from part II of this book into this routine to add variety.

Muscle group or region targeted	Exercise	Sets	Reps
Quads	Front squat	1	10
Hamstrings	Single-leg flexed-leg bridge	1	10
Glutes	Reverse hyperextension	1	12
Lower leg	Leg-sled calf raise	1	10
Quads	Single-leg squat	1	8
Hamstrings	Exercise-ball supine leg curl	1	10
Glutes	Step-up	1	10
Lower leg	Machine seated calf raise	1	10
Rest between exercises only as needed to maintain proper form.			

10-MINUTE LEG STRENGTHENER

Explanation   This time-saving routine will challenge you yet only take about 10 minutes. Take note that there is no equipment involved; therefore you will not have to put weights back or change settings on machines. You can also do this workout with very little space while traveling or at home.

Muscles Worked   Quads, glutes, hamstrings, adductors

Variations   Substitute any body-weight exercise from any category of exercises in part II of this book for variety.

Muscle group or region targeted	Exercise	Sets	Reps
Quads, glutes	Body-weight squat	1	10
Quads, glutes, adductors	Wide squat	1	10
Quads, glutes, hamstrings	In-place lunge	1 each leg	10
Quads, glutes, hamstrings, adductors	Lateral lunge	1 each leg	10
Quads, glutes, hamstrings	Retro lunge	1 each leg*	10
*Go to the top and repeat the sequence.			
Rest 10 to 20 seconds between exercises if needed.			

10-MINUTE GLUTE BUILDER

Explanation   This very simple routine will work your glutes and only take about 10 minutes.

Muscles Worked   Glutes, hamstrings, low back

Variations   For added resistance, you can keep the ankle weights on throughout the entire routine.

Exercise	Sets	Reps
Exercise-ball lying hip extension	1	12
Ankle-weight all-fours hip extension	1 each leg	12
Single leg bridge	1 each leg	10
Miniband lateral walk	1*	10 steps in each direction
*Go to the top and repeat the sequence.		
Rest 10 to 20 seconds between exercises if needed.		

10-MINUTE QUAD BUILDER

Explanation   This time-saving routine will work your quads hard yet only take about 10 minutes. Take note that there is very little equipment involved; therefore you will not have to put weights back or change settings on machines. You can also do this workout with very little space while traveling or at home.

Muscles Worked   Quads, glutes

Variations   To add extra resistance to this routine, hold dumbbells during the single-leg squats, exercise-ball squats, and in-place lunges.

Exercise	Sets	Reps
Front squat	1	10
Single-leg squat	1 each leg	10
Exercise-ball squat	1	10
In-place lunge	1 each leg*	10
*Go to the top and repeat the sequence.		
Rest 10 to 20 seconds between exercises if needed.		

10-MINUTE HAMSTRING BUILDER

Explanation   This hamstring time-saving routine will work you hard yet only take about 10 minutes. Take note that there is very little equipment involved; therefore you will not have to put weights back or change settings on machines. You can also do this workout with very little space while traveling or at home.

Muscles Worked   Hamstrings, low back

Variations   Substitute any hamstring exercise in this routine as long as it does not require a lot of time-consuming equipment changes.

Exercise	Sets	Reps
Double-leg straight-leg bridge	1	10
Hamstring lower	1	10
Single-leg toe touch	1 each leg	10
Exercise-ball leg curl	1*	10
*Go to the top and repeat the sequence.		
Rest 10 to 20 seconds between exercises if needed.		

10-MINUTE CALF BUILDER

Explanation
This very simple routine will work your calves hard and only take about 10 minutes.

Muscles Worked
Calves (gastrocnemius and soleus)

Variations
To add variety, consider exchanging a tibialis anterior exercise (heel walks, resistance-band inversion, and so on) for one of the calf exercises.

Exercise	Sets	Reps
Standing calf raise	1	10
Seated calf raise	1	10
Leg-sled calf raise	1	10
Machine seated calf raise	1*	10
*Go to the top and repeat the sequence.		
Rest 10 to 20 seconds between exercises if needed.		

Appendix

Metric Equivalents for Dumbbells and Weight Plates

The tables here provide conversions for common dumbbell and weight plate increments. For weights not listed here, you can calculate conversions using this equivalent: 1 kilogram = 2.2 pounds.

POUNDS INCREMENTS CONVERTED TO KILOGRAMS

Pounds	Kilograms
DUMBBELLS	
5	2.3
10	4.5
15	6.8
20	9
25	11.4
30	13.6
35	15.9
40	18.2
45	20.5
50	22.7

Pounds	Kilograms
WEIGHT PLATES	
2.5	1.1
5	2.3
10	4.5
25	11.4
35	15.9
45	20.5

KILOGRAMS INCREMENTS CONVERTED TO POUNDS

Kilograms	Pounds
DUMBBELLS	
2.5	5.5
5	11
7.5	16.5
10	22
12.5	27.5
15	33
17.5	38.5
20	44
22.5	49.5
25	55
30	66

Kilograms	Pounds
WEIGHT PLATES	
1.25	2.75
2.5	5.5
5	11
10	22
15	33
20	44
25	55

About the Author

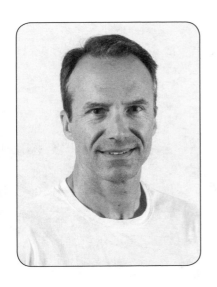

Tim Bishop owns and operates PerformFit, a sport performance and fitness facility, in Lutherville, Maryland. He also creates strength and conditioning programs for Ripken Baseball's summer camps and clinics. Bishop served as the strength and conditioning coach for the Baltimore Orioles for 14 years. He also played professional baseball for the New York Yankees and, as a two-sport star, took part in the NFL training camp in St. Louis.

He has appeared on numerous television and radio stations to promote health and fitness and is a frequent contributor to *Men's Health*, *Maximum Fitness*, and *Men's Fitness* magazines. His training advice has appeared in *USA Today*, the *New York Times*, and the *NSCA Journal*. He has lectured on a variety of topics for the NSCA, M-F Athletics, the Professional Baseball Athletic Trainers Society, and various colleges and universities. In addition, he is coauthor of the *Power for Sports* DVD (Human Kinetics, 2006).

Bishop has a bachelor's degree in human movement and sport studies and a master's degree in exercise science. He is a certified strength and conditioning specialist and a registered strength and conditioning coach through the National Strength and Conditioning Association.

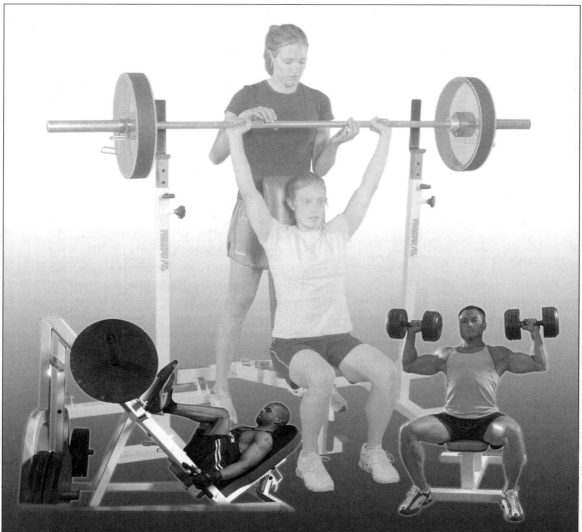